Charles Clark graduated in medicine from the University of Edinburgh and was appointed the youngest Consultant Surgeon in the UK in 1988. He is unique in achieving Doctorates in Medicine, Surgery and Science and, as a combined graduate in Medicine and Law, holds a judicial appointment and is a senior medical expert witness in medical legal disputes. As a recognised international expert on diabetes and glaucoma, he has published more than eighty scientific research articles in major peer-reviewed journals and is currently involved in nutritional studies in Glasgow and London. He holds an appointment as Clinical Research Fellow in Glasgow and has a private practice in London, with many high-profile patients.

Maureen Clark has been involved in the promotion of preventive health for many years, co-authoring eleven bestselling books on health and nutrition, published in sixteen countries and all still in print. Her last book, which sold over 100,000 copies worldwide, was specifically directed at young children to encourage healthy nutrition from the earliest possible age. She is a Fellow of the Society of Antiquaries of Scotland.

HEALTH
REVOLUTION FOR
MEN

Kick-start your weight loss and reduce your risk of serious disease – in 2 weeks

DR CHARLES CLARK

BSc, MB ChB, DSc, MD, ChM, LLM, FRCS, FRCOphth, FRACS, FRANZCO, FAAO, FIBiol, FAIBiol, FRMS, FRSM, FSAScot, CBiol

MAUREEN CLARK

FSAScot

piatkus

PIATKUS

First published in Great Britain in 2012 by Piatkus
Reprinted 2012 (twice), 2013

A CIP catalogue record for this book
is available from the British Library.

ISBN 978-0-7499-5349-2

Illustrations © Graham Gilhooley, zero7zero4
Designed and typeset in Albertina and Depot by Paul Saunders

Printed and bound in Great Britain by Clays Ltd, St Ives plc

Papers used by Piatkus are from well-managed forests
and other responsible sources.

MIX
Paper from
responsible sources
FSC® C104740

Piatkus
An imprint of
Little, Brown Book Group
100 Victoria Embankment
London EC4Y 0DY

An Hachette UK Company
www.hachette.co.uk

www.piatkus.co.uk

The information in this book, although based on the authors' extensive experience,
is offered as general guidance on the topics featured and is not intended to be a
substitute for the advice of your doctor. You are advised to consult your GP before
changing or ceasing any medication, medical treatment or medical advice.

Neither the publishers nor the authors accept any responsibility for any legal
or medical liability or other consequences which may arise directly or indirectly
as a consequence of the use or misuse of the information in this book.

This book is also available as an ebook

Contents

Acknowledgements

We would like to acknowledge the kind support and advice of Anne Lawrance and Jillian Stewart of Little, Brown, our steadfast – and patient – editors throughout the project. Margaret Wand, a Clinical Psychologist, provided invaluable insight into the male psychological approach to various situations. And, of course, our 'children', David and Heather (although at 20 and 17 years respectively, hardly children) have continued to provide forthright opinions on our work throughout the eleven books we have published on health and nutrition, which always improved the final manuscript and certainly entertained their parents!

Introduction

Life begins at forty. Actually life should be enjoyable at every
age but it can certainly begin to *end* at forty if you are not careful. However, in order to be able to enjoy life it is necessary
to slow the effects of ageing – and actually reverse many of
those already present, because most of the effects of ageing
are not permanent when we're in our forties and can be easily
reversed by lifestyle modification. Does this mean the aban-
donment of life to two hours of cardio in the gym? Certainly
not! It involves the development of a positive attitude and some
very simple and very easily implemented lifestyle changes that
can be achieved by everyone – at effectively no cost. The aim is to
promote health without drugs – wherever possible.

We have been engaged in the field of preventive medicine for
over twenty years and in that time there has been a 180-degree shift
in the approach of both doctors and men to the subject of men's
health. Previously, it was almost a taboo subject, hardly discussed
by men, as if it were some form of weakness to be anything but fit
and healthy. Even now, the 'macho' image still exists with many
men, but they are a dying breed – figuratively as well as actually –

and men are assuming an increasing interest in their own health, and, in so doing, changing their lifestyle to prevent many of the conditions of ageing.

What exactly are the conditions of ageing that we are proposing to reduce? The answer is virtually all of them, from heart disease and diabetes to obesity and arthritis! With only a few simple lifestyle changes? Within two weeks? Perhaps you find this difficult to believe but you will be convinced if you follow this simple programme. Of course, you can't reverse the changes of a lifetime in two weeks, but you will notice a substantial improvement in stamina and posture within that time – and you will begin to change shape significantly.

Although all of the major diseases can affect men and women, men are particularly susceptible to the following conditions:

■ heart disease

■ raised cholesterol

■ hypertension

■ diabetes

■ obesity

■ stress

■ back pain

■ loss of libido

■ and, of course, alcohol-related problems

A simple alteration in your diet can significantly reduce cholesterol levels – within two weeks – and therefore your risk of heart disease and hypertension. We are not suggesting you exist on salad and low-fat mayo (which doesn't work anyway) but enjoy delicious meals such as sirloin steak, chargrilled tuna, smoked salmon sashimi, duck breast with tarragon, chicken with chilli salsa, mushroom stroganoff, oven-baked ricotta with cherry tomatoes ... The potential combinations are literally unlimited. There is no calorie counting – on the contrary, the basis of this system is that you should never be hungry! How does it work? Quite simply, by altering the nutritional balance of your food intake, you will effectively programme your body to reduce body fat automatically. And all of the recipes are designed to be prepared simply, even by the most inept cook!

By following these basic principles you will also reduce your risk of diabetes – or improve your control of the condition if you already have it. Weight loss follows as a natural accompaniment to the loss of fat – without pain or effort.

Diabetes is increasing exponentially at present, with estimates predicting up to 24 per cent of the population having metabolic syndrome, which is the pre-diabetes condition. As diabetes is a major cause of heart disease, kidney disease, nerve disease and the commonest cause of blindness in the working population, it is definitely to be avoided. And it can be avoided in the majority of cases simply by a change in diet.

This initial part of the programme, which concentrates on diet, will result in significant improvements in health and appearance, but if you wish to obtain the full benefit, following the stress-reduction techniques we recommend will improve your heart-health even more. In many cases, it will also address the real underlying causes of loss of libido with advancing age. Stress is a major cause of most male health problems. All of the previously-mentioned conditions can be caused by stress, but there are many more: cancer, stomach ulcers, back pain and strokes all have stress as a major contributing factor. Reducing subliminal stress is remarkably simple, even in the most everyday stressful environment. It involves little time and can have major health implications. This programme includes simple yet highly effective techniques that can be employed in virtually every life-style situation to stabilise heart-rate, the single most important measure of general stress levels.

Another common problem for men over forty is a lack of

good posture and muscle tone, yet these are the foundation of preventing musculoskeletal problems such as back pain, arthritis, neck stiffness and muscular aches and pains. These problems can be substantially reduced by simple isometric exercises which can be performed in virtually any situation, without the need for expensive gym equipment. Isotonic exercise complements this essential core development, and a realistic programme for both types of exercise is featured in the text, along with helpful illustrations.

And finally, alcohol! Of course it's not an exclusively male problem but it can be a long-term one for many men and it needs to be addressed if you want real quality of life. Having said that, we do not advocate total abstinence; as you'll discover, the advice on alcohol intake in this programme is practical and effective, not proscriptive and ineffective.

We have treated thousands of men with problems ranging from the seemingly minor, such as obesity, to more major, such as raised cholesterol, diabetes and heart disease. In virtually every case there has been substantial improvement as a result of simple lifestyle changes alone.

Why don't you join them?

CHAPTER 1

Weighty Matters

For a long time it was assumed that men have a much easier time than women when it comes to body shape. After all, we hear a lot about the 'perfect' female body. However, while there are some elements of truth in this idea, the notion of 'perfection' is obviously wrong. From a psychological perspective, there's intense pressure on men, particularly those over forty, to maintain a 'healthy' body shape – not only for appearance's sake but because health seems to equate with how we look. While this is not entirely true, it is certainly a perception that causes significant psychological problems for men over forty.

However, before discussing body shape, we need to understand how it develops, and, much more importantly, how the paunch of middle-age spread can be removed.

There are basically three types of body shape for a man:

- The *ectomorph* is usually tall and slim.

- The *mesomorph* is commonly described as athletic and muscular, but is actually just the normal body shape with relatively small amounts of external body fat.

■ The *endomorph* is characteristically of larger proportions with a generous waist size – which is a subtle way of saying overweight.

These characteristic body shapes are a fairly accurate reflection of the subdivisions within the male population, although there are significant overlaps between them. However, it is important not only to *describe* body shape but also to explain *how* that body shape has been achieved, and how it can be adapted into a more acceptable outline. This is vital not only for physical health but also, much more importantly, for psychological health, because being either underweight or overweight can cause significant long-term psychological problems. The most important point is that irrespective of your shape, it can be changed relatively easily with simple lifestyle changes: diet, exercise and stress reduction.

Shapes and sizes

Let's look at the shapes in a little more detail to understand what the problems are, and to understand how they can be addressed. Obviously only one of these shapes will apply to you, so we suggest you concentrate on the one that's closest to your own.

Ectomorphs

Ectomorphs display typical characteristics. They:

■ have relatively thin shoulders

■ have lean muscle mass

■ are slim

■ have relatively flat chests

■ have thin frames

■ find it difficult to gain weight

These body types typically don't gain weight. Female ectomorphs are the envy of other women because they seem to eat large numbers of calories and don't get any heavier. But most males would rather have a much more masculine appearance and probably find it frustrating that, no matter how much they eat, they simply don't pile on the pounds. There are very significant medical reasons why this should be so, and we will discuss them in a few moments, and also look at ways to address this particular body shape.

Mesomorphs

Mesomorphs display what we might call the typical male structure, with wider shoulders and narrower hips. However, this may be a rather flattering description, because the majority of people don't have this particular build unless they work very hard at it. In fact mesomorphs are of a much more normal shape, with *slightly* wider shoulders and narrower waists, but can be dramatically enhanced by exercise and diet. Mesomorphs display the following characteristics:

- a defined muscle structure
- a more V-shaped body structure
- they gain fat more easily than ectomorphs do but less easily than endomorphs
- their muscle mass can be increased by exercise
- relatively trim bodies

The aim is for us all – irrespective of body shape – to strive for a more mesomorphic body structure, or, if possible, an *even more athletic* mesomorphic body structure. The surprising thing is that achieving this requires both diet and exercise, not exercise alone, which is a common misconception.

Endomorphs

The endomorph is the more typical body type for most men over forty. In other words, they're overweight. Fat gain is quick and simple. Body fat is deposited primarily around the waist and tummy with thinner arms and legs. That said, most endomorphs were actually rather more muscular in their youth, and, once again, with diet and exercise (more of the former) this enviable shape can be regained.

The typical traits of an endomorph are these:

■ They tend to be fat around the waist, much more so than the rest of the body.

■ They can increase fat quite quickly with relatively small amounts of food.

■ They have an underlying muscle structure that is dormant but can be re-enlivened.

■ They find it difficult to lose fat.

This is by far the commonest body shape in men over forty, but crucially it is also the easiest to change.

To understand *how* you can address this relatively easily with diet and simple exercise we need to understand how that fat accumulates.

The insulin dilemma

Body fat in a man accumulates around the waist and abdomen. The reasons for this are not as obvious as they may seem. Why doesn't fat accumulate in the rest of the body? Of course, if you are grossly obese then there will be fat around your arms, legs and chin, but in the majority of individuals this isn't the case, and their shape is more that of an apple. This is certainly not by chance. It occurs because of a very simple and straightforward medical process, as fat is deposited exclusively by a hormone called *insulin*.

Insulin deposits fat, from our food, around the waist. It's as simple as that. So, if we slow the production of insulin, the fat will disappear. It has nothing to do with calories or exercise, although these are important. It is simply a fact of life that if you reduce the body's production and level of insulin, the fat cells will disappear. In other words, insulin is the hormone that *makes* fat, and, as we reduce insulin, we *burn* fat. Nothing else.

So, if you intend to address the problem, you need to understand what makes insulin and how the process can be reversed. There are three main stimulants of insulin:

- refined carbohydrates

- stress

- certain types of medication

In essence, the cause of increased insulin production – which is the result of what we call *insulin resistance*, the phenomenon by which insulin becomes less able to reduce blood sugar – is too much carbohydrate, or 'carb', in the diet. Refined carbs cause insulin levels to increase, which lowers blood sugar (a state known as *hypoglycaemia*), and this stimulates our appetite to consume more carbs. Every cell

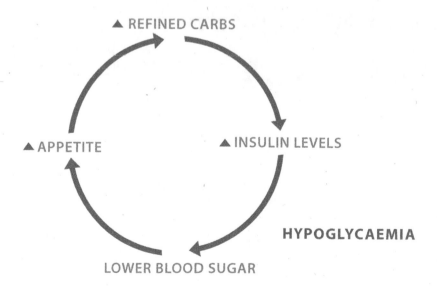

▲ REFINED CARBS

▲ INSULIN LEVELS

▲ APPETITE

HYPOGLYCAEMIA

LOWER BLOOD SUGAR

in the body has receptors for insulin on the surface of the cell. The more insulin you produce (in response to increased carb consumption), the smaller the number of receptors on the cells, therefore you produce even more insulin to compensate: it's a vicious circle.

The carbohydrate cycle

But what *are* carbohydrates? In simple terms, they're sugars – basically, sugar molecules joined to one another (see below).

There are two distinct forms of carbohydrate:

- *refined* carbohydrates, such as bread, pasta, rice, cakes, confectionary
- *unrefined* carbohydrates, such as vegetables and fruit

It is the *refined* carbs you have to eliminate if you intend to reduce insulin levels, and therefore lose fat, and hence change your body

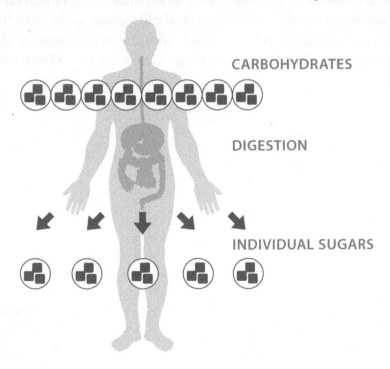

CARBOHYDRATES

DIGESTION

INDIVIDUAL SUGARS

shape. Refined carbohydrates have no nutritional value whatso-ever. There is effectively no nutrition in bread, pasta, rice, cakes, confectionary and processed foods. Of course, there is a little vitamin B in wholegrain rice but nothing significant. Most of these foods are actually 75 per cent carbohydrate, and therefore 75 per cent sugar because – and it is vital to remember this – carbohy-drates are simply converted to sugar within the body.

So if you eat, for example, a sandwich with two slices of bread, this is the equivalent of 40 grams of carbohydrate or 8 teaspoons of sugar in your body. This is absorbed from the bowel very quickly and you get a rapid energy boost. However, to counteract that, the body produces the insulin to lower the blood-sugar level. So we have the carbohydrate cycle.

But worse is to come: as your blood-sugar levels go up and down, you get variations in mood, concentration and irritabil-ity. When your blood sugar is high you are fairly stable; when it's low you become irritable, moody and experience low levels of concentration. And, as we have seen, when your blood sugar goes up, insulin causes the production of fat because insulin is the hormone that makes fat from blood sugar. So, if you can lower your blood sugar, and lower insulin production, you will then burn your body's fat, particularly from the place you most want to – around your waist.

To put it simply:

- when you are hungry, you eat refined carbohydrates, often in excess, which provide energy

- your body makes insulin to lower the blood sugar, but then the blood sugar dips too much and you need to eat more carbohydrates

- insulin converts the calories from carbohydrates into body fat, especially around the waist in a man

- and, even worse, the insulin prevents the body fat that you have being utilised for energy

INSULIN

CONVERTS EXCESS   PREVENTS THE BODY
CALORIES TO BODY FAT   BREAKING DOWN BODY FAT

The effects of insulin

When you reduce the insulin you will, in addition to reducing body fat, have much more energy, your waist will shrink in size, you will have much more concentration, and your mood swings will be fewer and less pronounced. Irrespective of the number of calories you eat, your waist circumference will decrease simply as a result of lowering insulin by dietary means. And, in reducing fat, you have switched on the body's fat-*burning* mechanism.

So how do you go about this? The secret lies in something called the *glycaemic index*.

What is the glycaemic index?

The glycaemic index (GI) indicates the rate at which foods are converted to sugar. High-GI foods are those that are high in sugar content and lower in nutrition, such as bread, pasta and rice; processed foods such as pies and pastries, cakes and confectionery, chocolate and some cereals; and certain types of alcohol such as lager and beer. So, if you cut these foods out of your diet, you will inevitably lower your insulin level and will stop making fat and start burning it instead, as insulin prevents the utilisation of body fat for energy. Therefore, the less insulin you manufacture, the more body fat you will lose.

To understand how to lose the fat around your middle, and increase muscle mass simply from diet, you really have to understand the glycaemic index. It may seem very complicated, but it simply represents the extent to which any particular food raises or lowers the blood-sugar level.

Obviously, we have to have a standard with which this is compared, and the standard we use, as you may expect, is sugar. Sugar is awarded a glycaemic index of 100, so all other foods are compared to pure sugar. Sugar is absorbed into the bloodstream usually very quickly, and then rapidly converted into fat. The glycaemic index is the rate at which other foods are converted into sugar. You may be surprised at just how quickly that happens with some foods. For example, did you realise that bread, pasta and rice have a glycaemic index of about 73, which means that they are converted into sugar in the bloodstream at 73 per cent of the rate of pure sugar?

On the other hand, natural foods such as meat, eggs, cheese and vegetables have the lowest glycaemic index. Meat, eggs and fish (in fact all forms of animal protein) have a glycaemic index of zero. Therefore, these foods have very little effect on blood-sugar levels and hence very little effect on insulin levels. This means that when they form a major part of your diet they are guaranteed to cause you to lose fat around your waist.

In summary, foods can be categorised as follows:

High-GI foods

- bread products (including wraps, panini, ciabatta and tortillas)
- pasta (all varieties)
- rice (all varieties)
- processed foods
- cake, confectionary, biscuits
- pies and pastries
- chocolate
- breakfast cereals
- dried fruit

■ some alcoholic drinks, such as lager, beer, cider, sweet white wine, champagne

Medium-GI foods

■ fruits (especially banana, pineapple and mango)

■ pulses (beans, peas and lentils)

■ fruit juices

■ medium white wine (e.g. Chardonnay)

■ root vegetables (e.g. parsnips and carrots)

■ potatoes

■ dairy products (e.g. yoghurt, cream and milk)

Low-GI foods

■ all animal-based products, including poultry, beef, pork, lamb

■ eggs

■ cheese

■ fish and shellfish

■ pure fats including oils such as butter and olive oil

■ spices

■ herbs

■ most vegetables (exceptions are potatoes, parsnips and some other root vegetables such as carrots)

■ tea

■ low-calorie soft drinks

■ artificial sweeteners

■ some alcoholic drinks such as whisky, gin, brandy, red wine, dry white wine

So the key to reducing that spare tyre round the middle and producing the mesomorph physique is to . . .

Reduce the insulin

By cutting out refined carbohydrates you will reduce your insulin levels, and therefore:

- you won't deposit fat on the waist

- you will actually *remove* fat from the waist by burning it

- you won't be weak and irritable due to hypoglycaemia (low blood sugar)

- you won't need to eat more carbohydrate, as reducing insulin reduces the need for more sugar

In other words, you will have broken the fat-creation cycle and your body will actually start to burn fat. You will have succeeded in switching off your body's fat-building mechanism, and switched on its natural fat-burning mechanism.

And the way that this is achieved is very simple. All you have to do is: *stop eating high-GI foods*.

So, with one simple action, you will not only stop making fat, but you will start to reduce the fat around your waist while not reducing calories or doing any exercise. This does not mean that exercise is not of great benefit, it certainly is, but for very different reasons, which I will outline later. As you can see then, losing the fat around your waist does not relate to reducing calories, but actually changing the *type of food* that you are eating. Indeed, the number of calories has no relevance to this whatsoever. With an identical calorie intake, a high-GI diet will put weight on and a low-GI diet will take it off.

In very simple terms (and at the risk of sounding repetitive), refined carbohydrates are high-GI, and therefore liable to cause weight gain; fats and proteins are low-GI and therefore guaranteed

IDENTICAL CALORIE INTAKE

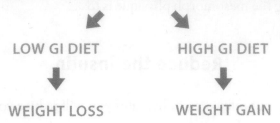

to cause weight loss. Yes, it seems remarkable that you can eat fats yet lose fat from your body, but that is a fact of medicine.

We'll look more closely at the food you eat in Chapter 10, 'Improve Your Food Awareness'.

For now, let's look at some of the successful results that have been achieved with this approach.

CASE HISTORY • ALEX

Alex was a forty-seven-year-old administrator who led a very sedentary existence. He embraced the typical office lifestyle: breakfast on the run, caffeine-fuelled day, office cakes, pub lunches, sweet snacks in the afternoon, then home for a takeaway after a long commute.

He had been recently diagnosed with type-2 diabetes, which was a shock to him. After all, as he reasoned, he was only forty-seven. At 5 foot 9 inches (1.75m), he weighed in at an excessive 84kg and had both raised insulin (12.6; normal is 5) and raised sugar levels (6.9; normal is 5.8).

He realised he had to change his lifestyle dramatically if he was to avoid a life on medication and multiple medical appointments. Following advice on the correct regime, he embarked on a low-GI diet, started taking →

light isometric exercise and set aside time – on a daily basis – to relax and de-stress.

The results were amazing. Within two weeks he had reduced his weight by 3kg, and in a further two weeks he had lost 4 inches from his waist measurement, and a whopping 9kg in weight. His insulin had reduced from 12.6 to 4.9 (normal), blood sugar levels had returned to normal at 4.9, and he had discontinued all diabetes medication. His only complaint was having to have all suits altered to fit his new shape!

CASE HISTORY • ALASTAIR

Alastair is a sales executive of a major company. His life consisted mainly of driving long distances to stressful meetings and ever-increasing sales targets. The stress and long hours made him constantly fatigued and the obligatory business lunches and dinners were taking their toll, as was the excessive alcohol intake, leading to a gradually increasing paunch. He had no time – or energy – for any form of exercise. Weighing in at an initial 105kg and with cholesterol of 7.3, he was heading for a heart attack.

His weight reduction after two weeks on this programme was 4kg and at the one-month mark his weight had reduced to 95kg and his cholesterol was down to 6.5. He had readjusted his eating habits to take advantage of healthier options rather than the quick fast-food fix. He had more energy, and was well on the way to recovery.

SUMMARY

▶ There are basically three essential body shapes: ectomorph, mesomorph and endomorph.

▶ The typical male shape after the age of forty is the endomorph, particularly with fat deposited around the waist.

▶ Fortunately, this is the easiest body shape to alter with appropriate dietary changes.

▶ Body fat around the waist is deposited largely as a result of the hormone insulin.

▶ Insulin levels are primarily raised by high-GI foods (such as refined carbohydrates) and, to a lesser degree, by stress. You can reduce insulin levels by reducing refined carbohydrates.

▶ Carbohydrates (or carbs) are merely sugar molecules joined together; carbohydrates are sugars.

▶ The glycaemic index, or GI, is a measure of the rate at which foods are converted to sugar in the body.

▶ Refined carbohydrates (such as those found in bread, pasta and rice) have a very high GI.

▶ To reduce body fat, particularly around the midriff, reduce insulin levels by eliminating (for a period only) all high-GI foods.

▶ For successful weight loss, and redistribution of body fat, forget calorie-counting and concentrate on a diet based on low-GI, high-protein foods.

CHAPTER 2

Protect Your Heart

Heart disease is the major killer of men in their forties and fifties. That's not a very pleasant prospect, but it is absolutely essential to consider these matters when you are in your forties or before, in order to prevent matters developing later in life – or to reverse a situation that may already be in the process of developing. The crucial points to bear in mind with heart disease are, first, that it usually develops over a period of many years, and, second, that it is preventable in the majority of cases. There are some individuals who, unfortunately, for genetic reasons, will develop heart disease to some degree no matter what they do. However, they make up a relatively small proportion of people with heart disease, since it is almost always caused by lifestyle factors – and not the lifestyle factors you might expect.

Most people think of heart disease as being restricted to the heart, when people have heart attacks or experience abnormal heart rhythms. However, heart disease is almost always *not* an isolated condition restricted to the heart, but rather a manifestation of generalised cardiovascular disease.

What does this mean? The cardiovascular system is made up of arteries (which take the blood with oxygen and nutrients to the tissues) and veins (which bring the blood back to the heart to receive more oxygen from the lungs).

This seems like a relatively simple system, and it is simple. However, it is also susceptible to conditions that affect the blood vessels. So, when we talk of heart disease, we are really talking about generalised cardiovascular disease, where all of the blood vessels are affected.

In essence, this means that, when you develop a narrowing or disease of the arteries, all the body's tissues are affected. When you have narrow arteries, for instance, the blood flow to various tissues is insufficient; therefore not only do you feel weaker with generalised tiredness (because the blood is not supplying the muscles well), but also every tissue in the body will be affected: the liver, heart, kidneys, the intestines and the brain. So the functions of all of these individual essential organs gradually deteriorate – the process we know as ageing.

Now obviously it is impossible to prevent ageing, as we will inevitably grow older, but we can certainly slow the effects of ageing by making appropriate lifestyle changes. Improving your health over a period of time is relatively simple: make sure that your body receives a good supply of oxygen and nutrients from food and the tissues will remain healthier for longer. The main cause of lack of nutrition getting to the body's tissues is actually narrowing of the arteries, preventing the life-preserving blood flow to the body.

If for any reason there is narrowing of the arteries, then obviously the blood carrying the oxygen and nutrition just can't get to the tissues and they gradually die. These processes tend to begin in men in their forties – or even thirties – and this is the time you can really make a big difference by staying healthy and preventing the development of lifestyle diseases, particularly heart disease, which can start to develop seriously in your fifties if you are not careful.

The major causes of narrowing of the arteries

The major causes of the narrowing of your arteries fall into three main categories: smoking, stress and your cholesterol level. Let's deal with each in turn.

Smoking

Smoking causes narrowing of all the arteries of the body and therefore prevents the cells receiving the food and oxygen that they need. Even apart from all the other diseases associated with smoking, such as lung cancer and various respiratory conditions, it undoubtedly accelerates ageing and the deterioration of all the cells of the body, so it is best avoided.

Stress

As we'll see in Chapter 3, 'Chill Out', the body's stress system comprises hormones (which are chemical messengers) such as cortisol, and a part of our nervous system called the *autonomic nervous system*. Stress can cause a narrowing of the arteries and prevent blood getting to the tissues, therefore causing them to age and die. The autonomic nervous system – the largely unconscious mechanism

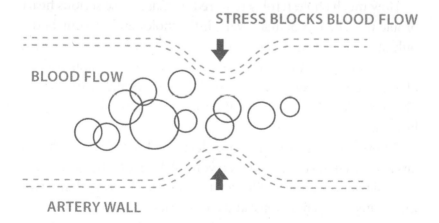

STRESS BLOCKS BLOOD FLOW

BLOOD FLOW

ARTERY WALL

that controls many body functions such as heart rate and digestion – affects every artery in the body. When we are stressed, it sends out signals that cause the arteries to constrict.

Cholesterol

Much is written about cholesterol and the importance of lowering *blood* cholesterol, but what exactly is this and how does it develop? And, much more importantly, how can we prevent cholesterol from clogging up our arteries?

Cholesterol is a fat in your blood that is largely produced by your own liver – 85 per cent of blood fats, in fact, with the remaining 15 per cent coming from food. So most of the advice you have been given regarding avoiding high-cholesterol foods is incorrect. How can this be proved? Very simply, really. The notion that high-fat foods provide high levels of blood fats is based on the principle that fats (in your diet) cross the bowel wall into the bloodstream. True. So far, so good. But the next stage – that these blood fats are then transported back to the heart by the veins – is wrong.

The blood from the bowel (full of carbohydrates, fats, proteins, minerals, vitamins and water) is transported to the liver, processed there, *then* goes back into the normal venous blood on its way back to the heart. So it is instantly apparent that it is the liver that filters the fats from the blood – and the liver that makes blood fats.

How much cholesterol is required to cause these serious heart problems? There is actually very little cholesterol in your body: only about 150 grams (5¼ ounces), of which only about 7 grams (a quarter ounce) is actually in the bloodstream. Yet the 7 grams in the bloodstream can cause narrowing of the arteries and heart disease. The next obvious question is: if cholesterol causes heart disease, how can you lower it?

Before answering that question, let us look at the various blood fats to understand them, and then you will be in a better position to control your own health. Blood fats are basically divided into two main categories: cholesterol and triglycerides.

As we have seen, 85 per cent of the fats in your blood are made in your own liver, and don't come from food.

Triglycerides are very bad: they clog up the arteries and are the major cause of heart disease, so it is absolutely essential to lower them (and, as you will see, this is remarkably simple).

Cholesterol is divided into two main categories, one that is protective and the other not so (you sometimes see them referred to as 'good' and 'bad' cholesterol):

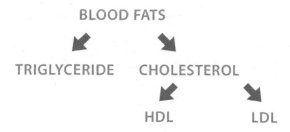

- *high-density lipoprotein* (HDL) is the form of cholesterol that actually clears your arteries and keeps them healthier

- *low-density lipoprotein* (LDL) is a form of cholesterol that causes blocking-up of the arteries

So, if you want to remain healthy, the obvious solution is to increase your HDL (which clears the arteries), reduce the LDL (which blocks the arteries causing heart disease), and, most importantly, reduce the triglycerides. How can this be achieved? Well the obvious solution (and that proposed by a number of authorities) is to reduce the fat in your diet and follow a low-fat diet. This seems logical and would involve avoiding meat, most fatty fish, most dairy foods, most oils, most cheeses . . . In fact most of what you would like to eat.

The problem is that many people have followed this diet for more than thirty years now and the rates of heart disease are increasing,

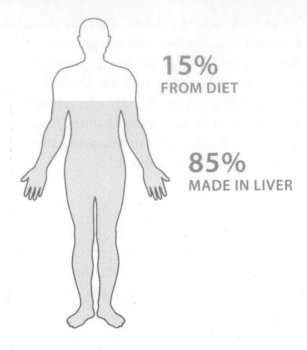

15%
FROM DIET

85%
MADE IN LIVER

SOURCES OF CHOLESTEROL IN BODY

not decreasing. In fact, there is strong evidence that a low-fat diet can actually *increase* triglyceride levels and reduce the HDL levels (which increases the risk of heart disease). So, in general, the low-fat diet is certainly not the answer to reducing heart disease.

If we consider the way that the body absorbs and metabolises the fat in your diet, this is exactly as you would expect. As already explained, 85 per cent of the cholesterol in your blood originates from your liver, not from your diet. So the question is: what causes this cholesterol and these triglycerides to be produced? The answer is sugar.

This seems absolutely crazy: how can sugar cause an increase in blood fats and heart disease? That's very simple to explain.

Let's go back to the 85 per cent of blood fats originating from your liver as a starting point. The triglycerides and the HDL and LDL from the liver are in fact controlled by *insulin*. Insulin is, once again, the villain, and insulin (as you recall) is primarily stimulated by refined carbohydrates such as bread, pasta, rice, cakes and confectionary.

Since, as we have seen, carbohydrates are merely sugars joined together, we could remove the word 'carbohydrate' from the language and replace it with 'sugar'. For example, bread, pasta and rice are made up of about 73–75 per cent carbohydrates (read 'sugar' when the carbohydrates are broken down into their constituent parts in your body). A slice of bread is the equivalent of about 4 teaspoons of sugar, and a banana is the equivalent of about 8 teaspoons. The point is that there are many hidden sugars in your diet that cause both insulin and blood fats to rise.

The obvious corollary is that the secret to reducing blood cholesterol is to reduce your intake of refined carbohydrates and any form of refined sugar. Many studies have shown that a reduction of insulin correlates directly with a reduction of artery-blocking triglycerides and an increase in the so-called 'good' cholesterol, HDL.

When we have cholesterol in our arteries, which makes our blood that bit thicker, what does it do? Cholesterol infiltrates the artery wall, making it much narrower and preventing blood from passing certain areas. In other words, it causes a mechanical blockage of the artery, which can eventually block entirely. In the case of the heart, this causes a heart attack.

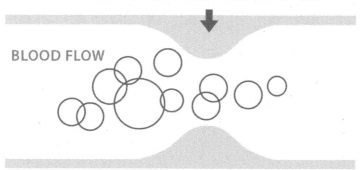

CHOLESTEROL BLOCKING ARTERY

BLOOD FLOW

ARTERY WALL

If there is narrowing of the arteries in other tissues, such as the liver and kidneys or in the arteries carrying the blood to the brain via the neck, this causes reduced function in all of these organs at the same time, so simply by reducing your cholesterol and triglycerides, you can improve the health of all of these tissues.

But those are the hidden advantages. The more obvious advantages are that when you increase blood flow to the muscles – including the heart – you will have much more energy and much less fatigue. Increased blood flow to the brain means that your mood will improve and your concentration will be sharper. So reducing cholesterol levels affects every organ in your body and will improve your standard of life immensely.

But this demon sugar doesn't only cause increased cholesterol and the blockage of arteries. It also accelerates the actual ageing process. Most of our structural proteins are made up of a building block called 'amino acids'. The amino acids join together and form the strong structural proteins from which bones, joints and muscles are formed. The bonds between the proteins need to be very tight because obviously there can be no points of weakness in bones or muscles.

But, if there is excessive sugar in the diet, the sugar molecules insinuate their way between the protein molecules causing them to be much weaker, and sometimes they can crack and break.

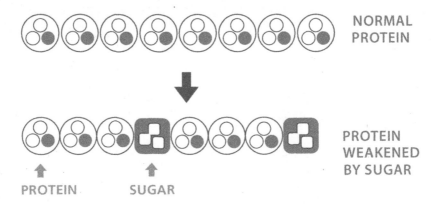

This infiltration by blood sugars into structural proteins causes weakening of bonds between proteins throughout the body, with rupture of small blood vessels, poor muscle function, weakened/brittle bones, and, most obvious, wrinkling of the skin. The medical term for this sugar problem is *glycosylation* and the actual sugars that cause the problem are called *advanced glycosylation end products*, or AGEs, which is a rather appropriate acronym for this process.

But, realistically, how effectively can you protect your heart? The following are examples of real men who have experienced the problems common to most of us. They changed their lifestyles and reversed their risk of heart disease.

CASE HISTORY • JAMES

James was a forty-one-year-old financier with a large investment bank. He had a major interest in maintaining his health and, in this context, trained regularly at the gym. Despite eating 'healthily' (he assumed) and frequently running marathons, he had steadily increased in weight by about 6kg over the previous six months. His occupation obviously involved a considerable amount of stress, and, although he did not smoke, he was very concerned about the possibility of future heart problems.

He realised there must be something intrinsically wrong with the advice he was following because, despite adhering rigidly to a diet and exercising regularly, he was still gaining weight. He decided to seek assistance. James weighed in at 85kg, which, for his height of 5 feet 8 inches (1.72m), was rather excessive. Much more concerning was a raised cholesterol of 7.1, providing a high risk of future heart disease, given his stressful occupation.

Once he instigated the recommended combination of effective dietary changes and stress-management techniques, he noticed an immediate improvement in energy and concentration levels. Within two weeks he had reduced his weight to 83kg and within one month his weight had decreased by 5kg to 80kg and his cholesterol measurement had dropped to 5.3. He had dropped one size in trousers from 36 to 34 inches, and had much more energy and stamina. In particular, he noticed his daily three-mile run was much easier.

CASE HISTORY • CONNOR

Connor was a forty-three-year-old lawyer, under considerable stress. Weighing in at 105kg with a height of 5 feet 9 inches (1.75m), he was very overweight, but of much more importance was his very elevated insulin level (a predictive factor for diabetes) at 17.6 (normal is 5). His cholesterol was 5.7 and he was finding it more difficult to continue with his hobby of cycling.

In essence, he was borderline diabetic with elevated cholesterol leading to potential heart problems in later life, despite not leading a sedentary lifestyle. He was a keen cyclist, cycling every weekend, but he was finding it gradually more difficult to maintain the energy required.

Stress and diet were the obvious problems to be addressed. When we identified the problem areas with lifestyle, he organised his daily timetable with the same care and application he applied to his profession, →

scheduling into his routine time to de-stress and replacing his fast-food lunches with equally fast *healthy* options. Late-night suppers became planned by having healthy alternatives rather than the convenient takeaway.

Within two weeks he had reduced his weight by 3kg and was achieving better cycling times. By four weeks his weight had reduced to 97kg (a reduction of 8kg), insulin levels had returned to normal at 6.1, cholesterol levels were back down to a healthy 4.6 and he was well on the way to recovery. His waist size had reduced by 2 inches and he was managing to cycle double the mileage in the same time.

SUMMARY

▶ Heart disease is just one manifestation of generalised blood-vessel disease throughout the body.

▶ Poor nutrition to the tissues – due to poor blood flow – can cause liver problems, kidney problems and memory problems, as well as heart disease.

▶ The main causes of blood-vessel disease, leading to heart disease, are smoking, stress and diet, particularly sugars in the diet, which raise the insulin level. Sugars in your diet increase your LDL cholesterol and triglyceride levels, and directly affect the development of heart disease.

▶ Heart disease can be prevented by not smoking, reducing stress levels (see Chapter 3: 'Chill Out') and reducing the level of refined carbohydrate in your diet.

▶ Most cases of heart disease can be prevented by simple adjustments to diet and nutrition.

Chill Out

Relax, reduce your stress levels and take it easier. This seems a very trite statement – because for many people that's easier said than done – but what really is 'stress'? You may think that stress simply means that we become a little agitated on occasions when adverse circumstances prevail. Isn't that it – end of story, problem solved?

So what is 'stress'?

Stress is the reaction that occurs in response to virtually every action of your body. And these actions are not under your conscious control. You are not in control of your body: your body is in control of you. You have no effective control over your heart rate, breathing, chemical reactions within your cells, sweating, changes in hair colour, bowel motions . . . The list is endless. All these essential bodily functions are the effects of the 'stress' mechanism. And this is controlled by two specific bodily systems:

- the stress nervous system, which is a very specific nervous system called the *autonomic nervous system*

■ hormones – which are chemicals that are transported in the blood – and specifically the hormone *cortisol*

This all seems a little technical but, if you consider for a few moments the way in which stress occurs, you'll realise that it becomes much easier to control it and prevent the medical conditions it causes.

The autonomic nervous system

The autonomic nervous system is a specific set of nerves that control the actions of every cell in your body. As you know, the spinal cord runs in the backbone and sends impulses (via nerves) to your muscles to control your voluntary actions. So, when you want to move your arm or your leg, you can voluntarily send a message from the brain, which travels down the nervous system via the spinal cord, and the muscle contracts.

But we don't consciously send nervous messages to control our breathing or our heart rate or the flow of blood in our arteries or all of the other many trillions of reactions that occur in the body every millisecond of every day. But they are still happening, so how does this occur? These actions are controlled primarily – but not exclusively – by the autonomic nervous system, which is entirely separate from the normal 'somatic' nervous system. This nervous system doesn't travel in the spinal cord but is situated on the front of the backbone and sends to all of the various organs and cells signals that control their actions. This nervous system is divided into two separate parts:

■ the *sympathetic* nervous system and

■ the *parasympathetic* nervous system

These nervous systems act in opposition to one another in every reaction of the body, so, when the sympathetic nervous system makes your heart beat faster, the parasympathetic nervous system makes it beat more slowly. Or, when the sympathetic nervous system dilates a pupil, the parasympathetic nervous system causes the pupil to constrict.

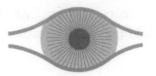 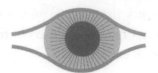

PARASYMPATHETIC
NERVOUS SYSTEM
CONSTRICTS PUPIL

SYMPATHETIC
NERVOUS SYSTEM
DILATES PUPIL

OPPOSING ACTIONS OF AUTONOMIC NERVOUS SYSTEM

So you can see that every action of the body is a balance between one function and the opposite reaction. Problems arise when one of these nervous systems becomes overstimulated and an imbalance occurs between them. So if, for example, you receive an unexpected surprise, the sympathetic nervous system has a much greater effect than the parasympathetic, and your heart beats much faster, resulting in such symptoms as:

■ dry mouth

■ pale skin

■ sweating

■ butterflies in the stomach

■ agitation

The chemical stress messengers

This is all very simplified of course. However, the second part of the stress nervous system is that controlled by hormones, particularly *adrenaline* and *cortisol*. When we receive a relative 'fright', which could be physical, emotional or psychological, certain organs in the body produce adrenaline and cortisol, and these cause similar symptoms to those of the sympathetic nervous system, such as dry mouth, dry skin, accelerated heart rate. This is part of the so-called *fight-or-flight response*, which was ideal for our hunter-gatherer forebears, who were fleeing from predators, but is not designed for the overreaction of the stress response in modern life, where our lifestyles tend to result in almost constant stress.

The adrenaline response may quickly recede but cortisol tends to remain in the system much longer and has much greater effects. The effects of cortisol are:

- increased blood pressure

- increased blood-sugar level

- decrease in the efficacy of the immune system

- decreased fertility

- decreased inflammation

The stress reaction is completely normal. A degree of background stress is essential for health, and the balance between the hormones and the nervous system is designed to keep us healthy. This is called *eustress* (i.e. good stress – the Greek word *eu*, meaning well, plus 'stress').

The problem arises when there is an imbalance between the stress nervous system and the stress hormones, or, much more importantly, when the stress levels remain too high for too long. This is known as *distress* – a very appropriate term. In other words, if our stress levels are elevated constantly, this causes distinct imbalances in the body and many of the medical conditions that will be described shortly.

Stress is probably the most serious condition that you will experience, because it causes so many different medical problems. Take the stress test. Do you suffer from any of the following at any time?

Abdominal paunch	yes/no
Anxiety	yes/no
Short temper	yes/no
Poor concentration	yes/no
Fast heart rate	yes/no
Hypertension (high blood pressure)	yes/no
Dry mouth	yes/no
Indigestion	yes/no
Constipation	yes/no
Regular colds/flu	yes/no
Back pain	yes/no
Fatigue	yes/no

If you scored 'yes' to between 8 and 12 of the above, your stress level is critical.

5–7: high stress level

2–4: medium stress level

0–1: I don't believe you!

But these are only *some* of the symptoms of stress, which can also cause:

- heart disease
- diabetes
- high cholesterol
- osteoporosis
- strokes
- some cancers

So you can see that stress doesn't really just involve 'occasional anxiety or being agitated', but actually has the potential to cause serious medical conditions. In order to understand this very complicated subject further and to prevent it from happening, we need to ask two specific questions:

■ What are the effects of stress and how does it harm you?

■ How can you prevent it?

Some solutions will be outlined as we discuss the causes and effects of stress in the following paragraphs, and then we'll move on to understanding the concept of time, effective de-stressing, control of the autonomic nervous system and the importance of effective breathing.

How does stress harm you?

Having seen the basic effects of our reactions to stress, let us look in detail at the medical conditions it causes and see just how dangerous it really is.

Abdominal obesity

Cortisol acts in opposition to the hormone insulin. As explained in Chapter 1, insulin is responsible for the production of body fat. In fact, it is the only hormone that controls body fat, so anything that acts against insulin will inevitably cause weight gain because the cortisol is preventing the insulin from being effective, so more insulin is produced. Net result: we put on more weight.

This is a vicious cycle: if the cortisol level remains high for long periods then insulin levels will remain high and the risks associated with increased weight will similarly increase. Much more importantly, as we've seen, insulin causes fat to be deposited around the lower abdomen in a male, causing the typical paunch.

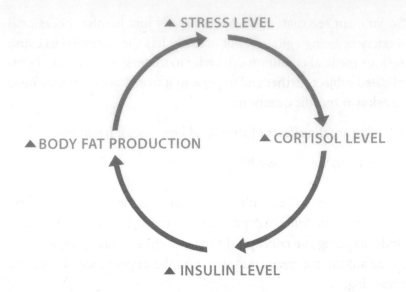

EFFECTS OF STRESS ON BODY FAT

And, if the insulin level is artificially elevated by insulin resistance (see 'The insulin dilemma' in Chapter 1) from an elevated cortisol level, then, crucially, it is impossible to lose weight from the paunch no matter how strict a diet you follow, because your body is working against you. And that is really the point: you simply cannot lose weight if your insulin level is high because of raised stress levels, so it is essential to control the stress levels to allow weight loss to progress.

Myocardial infarction

You don't normally expect serious heart disease to occur in your fourth decade, and hopefully not a heart attack, but the damage is usually beginning in your thirties, and by the time you reach your sixties the process is complete. The secret is prevention: halt the process of cardiac damage. This can be done, but before we get to that we need to understand the mechanism whereby heart disease develops. The heart is simply a muscular pump consisting of four chambers, which facilitates blood flow around the body to provide it with oxygen and nutrition. Each of the four chambers of the heart requires oxygen and nutrition, in the way all tissues have these basic needs, so there are obviously arteries leading to the heart that enclose the heart muscle.

This anatomical structure demonstrates the inherent weakness of the heart to external damage. These three arteries around the heart are the only supply of blood to the heart and therefore if they become damaged the heart is immediately affected, which can lead to a *myocardial infarction* or 'heart attack'. So your health is entirely dependent on three small arteries passing around the heart. And those arteries are subject to all of the potential problems that all other arteries encounter:

- narrowing and constriction

- blockage

- cell death

The main causes of blockage are:

- narrowing caused by stress from the stress nervous system

- narrowing caused by cholesterol

How does this constriction occur? When we become agitated (stressed) a nervous impulse is forwarded, via the sympathetic nervous system, to the artery and the artery constricts, reducing the blood flow (see artery on the right of the heart overleaf).

As the calibre of the artery is narrower, there is inevitably less blood passing through it (as with any narrow pipe) and therefore the muscle – the heart muscle – cannot obtain the oxygen and energy it requires, and cell death occurs. This problem is further compounded if the artery is already narrow due to blockage from cholesterol.

Cholesterol causes plaques to develop on the inner lining of the artery making it narrower, with a lower capacity for potential

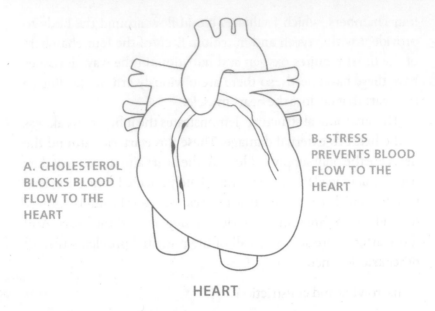

A. CHOLESTEROL
BLOCKS BLOOD
FLOW TO THE
HEART

B. STRESS
PREVENTS BLOOD
FLOW TO THE
HEART

HEART

blood flow (see artery on the left above). If we combine narrowing of the artery from stress with narrowing of the artery from cholesterol plaques, a heart attack occurs. On a positive note, both of these complications can be prevented.

High cholesterol

Raised cholesterol levels, although obviously associated with diet, are also significantly elevated as a result of stress. This leads to heart disease, hypertension (or raised blood pressure) and strokes, as raised cholesterol affects all of the arteries, and therefore prevention is essential. As we saw in Chapter 2, 85 per cent of the cholesterol in your blood originates in the liver in response to insulin. In other words, most of the cholesterol in your blood is not the result of a high-fat diet, but of insulin (which *indirectly* is dietary, because insulin is stimulated by sugar).

As we saw earlier, stress causes an increase in cortisol levels, which, in turn, causes an increase in insulin levels. Insulin, to a large degree, controls cholesterol levels, and therefore, if your

<pre>
      HIGH   HIGH
      CARB DIET   FAT DIET

          ⬇   ⬇

   ▲ INSULIN LEVEL   ▼ INSULIN LEVEL

          ⬇   ⬇

   ▲ BLOOD CHOLESTEROL   ▼ BLOOD CHOLESTEROL
     (FROM LIVER)   LEVEL
</pre>

EFFECTS OF DIET ON BLOOD CHOLESTEROL

cortisol level increases, by definition the fats in your blood will also increase. So cortisol causes raised cholesterol levels which, in turn, can lead to many diseases.

Diabetes

Diabetes is a condition where the blood-sugar levels rise and, if not adequately controlled, over a period of time cause damage to major organs in the body, primarily:

- impaired vision

- kidney dysfunction

- nerve damage

- heart disease

The problem is that high levels of stress can actually cause diabetes to develop. Once again, as we have already seen, stress causes the release of cortisol, and cortisol elevates insulin levels.

Elevated insulin is the first sign of pre-diabetes, and if this continues then diabetes will inevitably develop. So, if you are continually stressed, your cortisol levels will increase and, in association with its other many actions, it promotes the development of diabetes due to the constant elevation of insulin.

How common is diabetes?

That's really the problem. The prevalence of diabetes is increasing exponentially. At the moment, diabetes affects up to 8 per cent of the UK population, but the pre-diabetic state (called the *metabolic syndrome*) is estimated to affect up to 24 per cent of the population. So this is certainly not an uncommon condition. The last known statistic for the United States was 25 per cent. However, as that was in 1994, and the prevalence of diabetes has increased dramatically in the US since then, this percentage will undoubtedly be much higher today.

Hypertension

Hypertension means simply that the blood pressure is raised. The problem with raised blood pressure is that it can lead to:

- heart disease
- stroke
- dysfunction of all of the organs of the body

How does high blood pressure develop? There are several mechanisms, but the single most important one is undoubtedly stress. Stress causes constriction of the arteries and therefore it is harder for the heart to pump against these narrower vessels. The heart muscle has to work much harder, and so it enlarges in order to cope. The arteries around the heart cannot supply the heart with enough blood, and therefore the heart muscle begins to die – a heart attack.

Stress not only narrows the arteries making the heart work harder, it also narrows the arteries by increasing the cholesterol levels that block the arteries – a vicious circle.

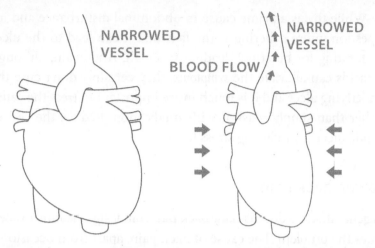

EFFECTS OF HIGH BLOOD PRESSURE ON THE HEART

Stomach ulcers

Ulcers in the stomach, or more commonly at the beginning of the intestine (called the duodenum), are almost exclusively associated with stress. The sympathetic nervous system causes the stomach to produce more acid and this wears away the lining of the stomach, causing an ulcer to develop.

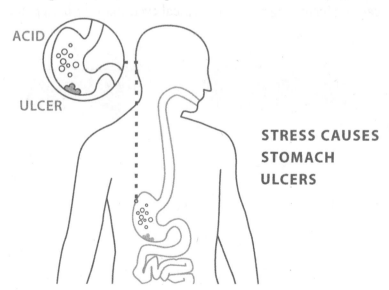

STRESS CAUSES STOMACH ULCERS

While this is a prime cause of abdominal disturbance and indigestion, more sobering is the fact that it can lead to the ulcer perforating (or bursting), leading to death. And again, although antacids can alleviate the *symptoms*, they certainly don't cure the underlying ulcer and it is much more important to treat the cause rather than simply mask it with medication. Reduce the risk of peptic ulcers by reducing stress levels.

Lower-back pain

In general, stress doesn't *cause* back pain, but it significantly exacerbates the problem. The cause of back pain, apart from occasional muscular damage, is almost exclusively a nerve being trapped between the vertebrae. The nerve is not usually trapped by the backbone itself, but rather by the discs between the vertebrae, which can rupture and compress the nerves.

When a disc ruptures, it bulges and presses on the nerve (usually leading to the lower back or the leg), and when it touches the nerve an intense pain reaction occurs. Unfortunately, as a result of the pain, the muscles around the disc go into spasm (see below), causing the bones to be pressed more firmly against the nerve and causing increasing pain – the typical cycle of lower-back pain.

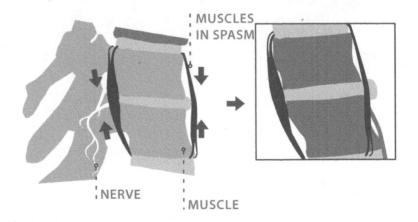

MUSCLES IN SPASM

NERVE

MUSCLE

MUSCLE SPASM IN BACK PAIN

The pain in turn causes more generalised stress in the body, and therefore the stress reaction is stimulated and the muscles contract even more in spasm, causing more pain. The standard treatment for lower-back pain is to rest for some weeks in bed, keeping the area warm and therefore reducing the stress reaction locally so that the muscles can relax and the disc can retract from the nerve, alleviating the pain.

So you can see that, although stress doesn't actually cause the initial back pain, it certainly exacerbates the problem and, if you can reduce the generalised stress, this will reduce the level of back pain. What you must not do is to simply try to 'mask' the pain by taking excessive amounts of analgesics (or painkillers), as these will not control the problem but merely hide it and therefore the underlying damage will continue.

Reduced immunity to infection

Cortisol reduces the body's natural immune system, which effectively means that, if you have an infection (typically of the chest), this can take much longer to cure, and even simple wounds take longer to heal. Stress increases cortisol levels and seriously reduces your immunity to infection.

Reduced libido

Cortisol also acts against testosterone, reducing libido significantly. Although the association between elevated cortisol levels and reduction in testosterone levels is well documented, how this happens is not known.

As if the above weren't enough, cortisol can also increase the risk of osteoporosis, and stress has been implicated significantly in the development of certain cancers.

As you can see, the effects of stress are not simply mild agitation and being emotionally unstable; it can cause many of the major medical conditions that, in turn, result in serious illness and potentially lead to death. It's impossible to overstate how important it is to reduce your stress levels at the earliest possible stage – at the latest by your forties and early fifties, otherwise permanent damage will occur.

How does stress develop?

As with all journeys, life's journey is full of expectations and end-points or goals that we wish to achieve. The problems associated with stress are often a result of our past experiences, and specifically, *how we deal with those experiences*. The important point about dealing with them, many of which are difficult parts of the normal learning curve of life, is most effectively expressed by Rafiki in *The Lion King*: after whacking Simba on the head unexpectedly, when he seemingly attempts this again, Simba avoids the blow and Rafiki excitedly shrieks that Simba has realised one of the most important lessons of life: *learn* from the past but don't *live* in the past.

Although you have no past experience at birth, experiences soon emerge, and we carry them with us throughout life. The problem is that experiences accumulate. We can't leave them behind. They gradually build up in our minds. The experience of life's journey is expressed in the way that we think, eat and behave, and it forms the basis of how we work, live and relate to others. These experiences are accumulated from our upbringing, education, friendships, other relationships and work. They have been compiled over time, learned and practised over years.

Some of life's experience gets ditched because it's not useful. Other parts are deliberately altered. But, unfortunately, most of your experience is retained, not because it is useful, but because it is remembered and is often difficult to eliminate. This relates to both good and bad experiences. However, unfortunately, the bad ones tend to be retained more, for reasons unknown. Much of this relates to inexperienced responses we have made in our early life, often under pressure. Many can be destructive, not only to you but to those around you. The question is: is it worth spending the time getting the best out of your life's experiences, and ditching the rest?

The best advice is probably to follow typical budget-airline baggage policy: *just carry on board what you need for the journey.* In other words:

■ take control of life's experiences, and use them to advantage – not disadvantage

■ manage stress by looking afresh at the different parts of your life

■ decide what are the things you really want to have realistically, rather than being guided by unrealistic aspirations

Remember the airline's advice:

■ you pay extra for travelling with excess baggage

■ excess baggage extorts a high price

■ excess baggage weighs you down

The stress that we experience basically originates from three main areas, and, more specifically, from three main experiences:

■ those of the past

■ those of the present

■ those of the future, which we anticipate we will experience

The human mind is a strange beast: it tends to dwell on negative thoughts rather than positive. When we think of the past relating to all of those experiences, there tends to be, in most individuals, a preponderance of negative thoughts in preference to their positive counterparts. We remember the negative effects and tend to carry those with us throughout life. This causes insecurity and anxiety, which can affect our daily lives.

In the present, it is important to realise that external events have an influence on everything you do. Every new job leads to changes and adjustments. Relationships have an effect on your life whether you have one or not. New corporate structures and cultures demand changes in how tasks are performed – even how you dress.

Work colleagues, relationships, friendships, neighbours all make emotional and psychological demands, which may be subliminal and not even realised. Most of the above appear to be beyond our ability to influence or control.

But the handling of change is actually totally under your control. It is just a question of deciding which changes are necessary and how to effect them. This may mean making adjustments to your lifestyle, possibly even downsizing in certain situations, but the pursuit of happiness and reduced stress is worth the effort.

Most of life consists of making knee-jerk reactions, repeating the usual responses, because we don't take the time for careful reflection. Financial and social pressures in general take precedence, but it's vital to think things through carefully, consider the options and make a balanced decision – rather than a hurried one that will probably result in even more stress.

Most of life's habits are rooted deeply in the past, responses that remain unchanged and are long past their sell-by date. Other behaviours are just reactions to situations, such as going to the fast-food outlet because it is nearer than a healthy alternative. The first thing to realise if you want to combat stress is . . .

Take your head out of the sand

Stress is the most damaging threat to a fulfilling life. It creates ripples far beyond the arena that causes the stress. It alters our physical shape, changes our diet, messes up relationships, damages friendships and, most importantly, makes us dislike ourselves – which, in turn, causes more stress. Only you will know which area causes you more stress, uses up your resources and leaves feelings of dissatisfaction and unhappiness – causing more stress. Unfortunately this leads to the chicken-and-egg dilemma:

- Where to begin?

- Will a happier home life improve my working performance?

- Will increased job satisfaction lead to better personal relations?

- Will feeling and looking better improve my self-esteem and other areas of life?

On days when such negative thoughts dominate and you feel as if you are being attacked from every side, you can employ 'stress elastoplasts'. This involves making space for yourself, but it need not be long. Researchers have found that reading something of real interest to you for as little as six minutes can reduce stress by 68 per cent. This stress buster is especially helpful as it is possible to use it almost anywhere. Other solutions are listening to music, which lowers stress by 32 per cent, or a weekly massage, which brings down the stress level by 27 per cent. However, all of these, albeit helpful, are merely elastoplasts. What you really need to do is identify and address the causes of the stress, not just alleviate the symptoms.

Understand the concept of time

Unless you can understand the concept of time and how to use it effectively and to your advantage, your attempts at controlling your stress are unlikely to be successful. Time is an intangible that has an inexorable progress – irrespective of any other aspect of life. You cannot control time. You cannot stop it and you certainly cannot reverse the march of time. It is there for you to use. The problem is that we have many constraints on our time that make it seem as though we are out of control. For example, for a typical man in his forties and fifties the three main constraints are:

- financial
- family
- leisure

These constraints need to be balanced to lower stress levels and reduce damage to the heart. Unfortunately, pressures such as financial and family can have major consequences on your management of time, and usually reduce leisure time to a minimum. Similarly, men who place too much emphasis on leisure time can experience family problems, a common cause of stress. The solution is to understand the *concept* of time and how it can be used to maximum advantage.

To date, only one group of people have been discovered who actually have no concept of time. In the Amazonian jungle, the Amondawa tribe, 'discovered' in 1986, have no understanding of the concept of time as an entity. There are no words for 'time', 'week', 'month' or 'year' in their vocabulary. They don't think of tomorrow but just of today. Although there is no data regarding whether this causes them to have less or more stress, the likelihood, on the balance of probability, is that there will be much less stress because they are not concerned about the future or the past but just about the present. And, at the end of the day, that is all that you can do, because the present is all you actually have.

These people live in a world of events, but they don't see those events as being embedded in time, because time does not exist. And, whether we like it or not, that is exactly what life is. Experiences do not exist in time because, when that time has passed, so have the events. We normally think of time as a distinct entity, with phrases such as 'I haven't got the time', 'It is time to go home' and 'The weekend is nearly over'. There is a common association between 'time' and 'finance', but this is a nebulous association. It is essential to accept that time isn't money, and, in the majority of cases, you don't need to race against the clock to achieve a certain status. Time is there to be utilised, not to utilise you, and unless you understand that basic concept then stress management will be impossible.

The problem of unsocial hours

Unsocial hours are an inevitable consequence of modern society. The type of job that requires you to work unsocial hours has spread beyond the traditional industrial fields of health, emergency services, transport and continuous-process manufacturing into supermarkets, airports, bars and more social activities.

While society runs twenty-four/seven, the human body is still operated by a body clock that expects sleep at night and that influences body temperature, alertness and appetite. These physical, mental and behavioural changes follow a twenty-four-hour cycle, responding to light and darkness in the environment. The human body clock synchronises temperature, heart rate, blood pressure and mental ability so that they are higher during daylight hours than at night and are at the lowest point about 3 a.m. It also regulates the immune system and is involved in the division of cells.

Fighting our internal body clock leads to complications. About 14 million people in the UK work unsocial hours; of these, about 66 per cent report some kind of ill health.

Compared with workers who have a 'normal' nine-to-five existence, those working unsocial hours are at higher risk of diseases such as obesity, cardiovascular disease, digestive problems and failure to control blood-sugar levels. At least some of these may be linked to the quality of the diet and irregular timing of eating.

These health problems are aggravated in the short term by fatigue, loss of concentration, a higher rate of absence from the job and poor sexual performance. Factors that may play a part include stress, disrupted body rhythms, sleep debt, physical inactivity and insufficient time for rest and revitalisation.

Taking control

Whatever the reason for your working unsocial hours, the consequences are the same: increased likelihood of eating at irregular times and consuming high-fat, high-calorie foods accompanied by 'energy' drinks (high in caffeine) in order to stay awake.

Unsocial hours affect all bodily systems, particularly digestion. The digestive system slows down greatly at night because it expects the body to be asleep. Therefore, what you eat is of more importance at night than during the day. This is not about deprivation: it is about consuming foods that energise.

Eating well

Unsocial hours may mean you can't control *when* you eat but you can control *what* you eat – by planning and forethought. Here are some tips:

- Establish a normal meal schedule of three meals at regular intervals.
- Always start your day – whenever that may be – with protein.
- Remember that eating fatty or sugary foods gives a short-term boost but long-term illness.
- Avoid highly processed foods as they increase feelings of tiredness and lethargy.
- Minimise health risks by cutting out fast food.
- Snack on nuts and raw vegetables.
- Drink plenty of water.

Perchance to dream

Sleep is something else that unsocial hours can get in the way of. We all need a period of sound, undisturbed sleep to maintain health and wellbeing, whatever our working hours. The shortage of good-quality sleep often leads to chronic fatigue. This is harmful to all aspects of daily life.

Lack of sleep is demonstrated by irritability, tiredness and depression, not responses that make for happy families or warm friendships. Those who are always tired tend to suffer from loss of appetite and digestive problems.

Social consequences

Working unsocial hours often leads to being disassociated from family and friends, which can cause friction in relationships. Recognise that efforts need to be made by both sides to get the best out of this situation.

A little quiet discussion *and* listening on both sides can improve the quality of everyone's life. Understand that working hours and sleep patterns may leave partners feeling that all the responsibility of meeting family demands lands on them. Acknowledge the strains and explore any options to make family life less difficult.

Working unsocial hours on a regular basis inevitably leads to irregular patterns not only of work but of eating, sleeping and socialising that may also cause health problems. The most important requirements from a human point of view are that loss of sleep should be as little as possible, and to ensure there is sufficient quality time for family and social contact.

Be realistic about your life

- Recognise that no job, no relationship and no way of life is perfect, but it can be made more tolerable.
- Know that almost every situation can be improved.

Your current situation is almost certainly the outcome of unconscious 'drift'. In other words, you have probably allowed circumstances to dictate your life rather than taking control of the circumstances. Think in terms of *gradual development rather than radical change*: introduce changes slowly to adapt to circumstances rather than trying to change everything at once, which is a certain recipe for disaster. For example, don't be caught in the 'cereal for breakfast' trap: eggs are much healthier and just as quick and easy as cereal. But the adjustments have to start with you. Reduce your stress levels by taking control of the different aspects of your life.

What are the risks of challenging the status quo?

Challenging the status quo is always a risk. But it is usually much more of a mental risk than an actual risk. The types of pressures that are on us are emotional and financial, and these tend to encourage the *prevention* of change. Above all, risk involves serious emotional concerns and anxiety, which can lead to more stress.

Risk involves the freedom to:

■ try new ventures and accept the possibility of failure

■ have a positive attitude to change

■ accept mistakes at their face value, and not as a sign of failure

■ accept change as part of life

■ go for improvement and don't worry about failing

■ discuss ideas that may on the surface appear ridiculous and don't worry about being ridiculed

■ focus on now and not on the future

Although it is often trite to give quotations, undoubtedly the most appropriate in this respect is that of Franklin D. Roosevelt in the depression of the 1930s when he said, 'The only thing we have to fear is fear itself.' This is true, and once accepted it can change everything. Fear of failure and fear of rejection cause more stress than probably any other subjects. They encompass all aspects of our life, from working environments and personal relationships, to taking risks that are by no means certain to be successful. But fear has to be confronted if you want to reduce your stress levels and achieve a healthy and more fulfilling life.

How to de-stress – effectively

So, having established how mental stress can have serious physical effects on the body, let us examine how to address this and prevent it from happening. As I've already said, there is no point in being influenced by events in the past, as the past is in the past. However, this is easier said than done, because we all carry mental baggage that travels with us throughout our lives. The answer is to ditch that baggage.

Similarly, there is no point in worrying about the future, as there may not be any future. No one can predict what will happen and many unfortunate individuals have planned for a future to find that unforeseen events ruin their plans.

So we are left with the present. And that is what we must concentrate on – not some nebulous event in the past that has affected us but can have no further relevance, and certainly not potential events in the future that may not occur. In fact, the most effective way of ensuring a happy future, however long that may be, is to concentrate on the present.

The second principle to emphasise is that, if you do really seriously intend to reduce your stress levels, you need to set aside time for this specific purpose on a regular basis. No amount of de-stressing techniques (such as music, CDs, relaxation programmes) are of any value unless you make a definite commitment on a regular basis. Of course, this is very easily avoided, like the gym membership that is never used after the first month. But the problem is that, unless you do actually set aside time on a regular basis to address the stress issue, it will not go away and the anticipated medical problems will inevitably occur.

What does this mean? It requires setting aside five minutes for yourself every day, irrespective of your daily commitments. It is all very easy for us to claim that we are far too busy and that other matters take up our time, but everyone has five minutes each day that they can set aside for themselves. Without this commitment, your stress levels will not be addressed and health problems will inevitably follow.

Controlling the autonomic nervous system

In order to control stress you need to control your autonomic nervous system. As we discussed previously, this is the nervous system that controls all of the everyday actions over which we seemingly have no voluntary control: breathing, heart rate, sweating, body temperature and so on. But, that said, we can actually exert a tremendous amount of voluntary control over it – with practice. Most of the actions of the autonomic nervous system are very difficult to measure but the most obvious is heart rate. And, contrary to popular misconception, it is not the *rate* at which your heart beats that is important but rather the *regularity*. Most people consider a slow heart rate to be healthy and a fast one unhealthy. In some regards this is true, but of much more importance is the *changing* heart rate rather than the rate itself. In effect, you are trying to achieve an even heart rate without changes from fast to slow.

In stress reactions, what happens is not that your heart rate increases and remains high all the time, but rather that it varies dramatically between faster and slower within fractions of a second (see diagram opposite, top).

When the heart rate is regular, all of the autonomic reactions in the body are coordinated, so by controlling one function you can control them all to some degree. The 'control centre' for your heart rate (along with breathing, sweating and many other functions) lies in a very tiny area called the *brainstem*, which is at the base of the skull. All of these areas are close together and coordinate very closely (see diagram opposite).

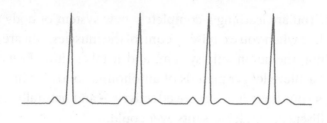

STABLE RESTING HEART RATE

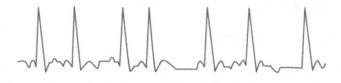

STRESSED HEART RATE

Strange as it may seem, to control your heart rate you do not concentrate on the heart rate itself but rather on the elimination of *negative conscious thoughts*. So how do you go about this?

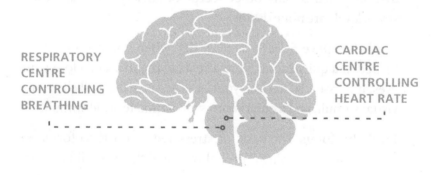

RESPIRATORY
CENTRE
CONTROLLING
BREATHING

CARDIAC
CENTRE
CONTROLLING
HEART RATE

Autonomic manipulation – the natural way to de-stress

The principles that you can follow to relieve stress are relatively simple. However, in practice, it takes time to see results and it is important to realise that even small achievements are a major success. You are learning a completely new system of body control. Unlike when you exercise to control the muscles, you are now controlling the autonomic system, and it takes time. Every day you will achieve longer periods of autonomic control, which will de-stress your body much more effectively – and naturally – than tranquillisers or antidepressants ever could.

De-stress exercise

Before you start, follow these tips:

- **Find the time** You need to devote at least five minutes – and preferably two periods of five minutes – set apart during the day, away from external stimuli, in peace, and you must be prepared to concentrate on eliminating all stimuli from your existence. This effectively resets the body's automatic systems and is most clearly exemplified by Buddhist monks who set aside long periods for the practice of meditation; in so doing, they achieve stable heart rhythms, which have never been demonstrated by any other sector of society. In effect, their stress levels are nonexistent.

- **Find the space** Select a time of day when you can be undisturbed in a quiet room. Sit in a relaxed manner and close your eyes. It is essential to close your eyes because this will eliminate visual stimuli, and a quiet room will eliminate aural stimuli.

- **Find the focus** The basis of stress reduction is to focus on *nothing*. Doing nothing is probably one of the most difficult exercises that you will ever attempt, and certainly one that you will not successfully achieve for quite some time. So don't expect immediate results, but, if you continue to commit to practice, you will be successful and stress levels will reduce.

- **Banish negative thoughts** As you probably realise, meditation is designed to eliminate all negative thoughts from the mind. As our minds are constantly active and generating thoughts of many different forms (unfortunately, many of them negative), to eliminate thoughts and external stimuli from all your senses is something that, in the initial stages, will occur for a few seconds, and later will become more effective. It is of absolute importance to eliminate thoughts during this process, as most thoughts are negative and are potent causes of more stress.

Now you are ready to begin.

1. **Concentrate on your breathing** Breathe deeply and evenly, trying to achieve a rate of about six to eight deep breaths per minute. This is quite difficult to achieve as usually our breathing rates are much higher than this and even concentrating on the breathing rate disturbs your elimination of all conscious thought.

2. **Concentrate on your heart** Now focus on your heartbeat. Although we have emphasised the need to focus on nothing, that is almost impossible, and to achieve this we need to focus on some bodily function over which we have no obvious control. What we are actually trying to achieve is to purge the traumas of normal life from our systems for a short time. So concentrate on your heart rate. Concentrate fully on the heart and think of absolutely nothing else. Although it's difficult to achieve initially, with time you will be able concentrate exclusively on your heart, which will eliminate all other thoughts. Try to continue this manoeuvre for at least two minutes – which is a very long time to clear your mind of negativity.

3. **Return to your breathing** Now transfer your thoughts to the rate of breathing. Concentrate on breathing slowly and evenly (at about six to eight breaths per minute, each cycle including both inhalation and exhalation) but do not count the rate. The reason for concentrating on breathing is that the breathing rate actually has a significant effect on calming all of the autonomic actions, including the heart rate. When you achieve even breathing without negative thoughts, the heart rate

gradually stabilises. It not only slows, but the variation in heart rate between fast and slow becomes very low. You can check this by taking your pulse at the time of the exercise. To take your pulse, simply place the fore- and middle fingers of your right hand on the left wrist, as shown below. As you breathe in, your pulse rate increases; as you exhale slowly the pulse rate decreases. This is the normal effect of the autonomic system on your heart.

4. **Banish those negative thoughts again** Concentrate on breathing very slowly and try to eliminate all negative thoughts. If necessary, think of positive thoughts in your life but preferably try to think of nothing at all. You will find this is extremely difficult at first, as the brain will inevitably be constantly trying to reintroduce thoughts and emotions, which have a significant effect on stress reaction. But, each time the mind returns to a conscious thought, try to eliminate it by focusing on emptiness. After about another two minutes, open your eyes and slowly reconnect with the outside world, once again trying to eliminate all negative thoughts of problems that you expect to arise in the future, as this only leads to a return to the stressful baseline.

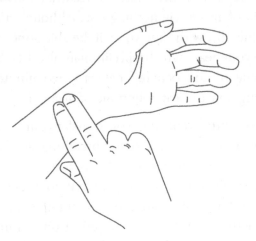

TAKING THE PULSE AT THE WRIST

As you will discover, this is a difficult exercise, and for some it may be impossible to achieve for more than a few seconds at a time initially. Don't be put off. As the months progress, you will find that relaxation is gradually improving and you will become calmer and less agitated. This is the simplest and least technologically complicated way of controlling stress. However, for those technologically minded, it can certainly be achieved visually by employing a positive feedback of your control of the autonomic nervous system.

Stress can be quantified – and controlled – by measurement of the variations in the heart rate using a computer-based programme called Heartmath, which enables you to develop a positive feedback of how your heart rate is progressing. The visual stimuli involved use a 'traffic light' system of red, amber and green, relating to high stress, medium stress and low stress. The basis of the programme is that when your heart rate's variability is very high – in other words the transition between fast heart rate to slow heart rate is occurring in milliseconds – then you are under high stress. Similarly, as the heart-rate variability decreases, this is a very accurate measure of the stress reactions coming under conscious and voluntary control.

When you actually see the results of your control over heart-rate variability demonstrated in this way, it can form a very positive reinforcement. The programme uses a small handheld monitor, or an external heart-rate monitor, which is connected via a computer to a simple sensor attached to your forefinger (see page 56).

You can then watch the lights on the monitor and, as red turns to green (once again, usually over a period of months rather than days), you have positive feedback that control of the autonomic nervous system is occurring. However, such technology doesn't come free, and is not necessary in view of the fact that the same result can be achieved without it.

Other approaches for reducing stress may involve exercise, listening to music or even using meditation CDs. While these are undoubtedly effective to some extent, they can control stress only to a certain degree because, unless negative thoughts are eliminated for periods entirely, there is a subliminal level of stress at all times.

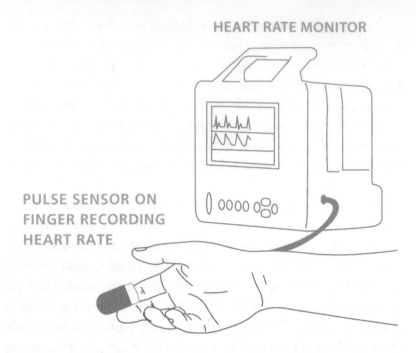

HEART RATE MONITOR

PULSE SENSOR ON
FINGER RECORDING
HEART RATE

The importance of breath control

Controlling breathing is the key to controlling stress. Breathing is
unlike any other function of the body, as it is the only function
that is under both *conscious control* and *unconscious (autonomic)
control*. You *can* consciously control your rate of breathing, but only
with a specific conscious effort; most of the time, you will breathe
at a rate of approximately twelve to eighteen breaths per minute,
without being consciously aware of this fact, because it is under the
control of the autonomic nervous system.

How does this relate to the control of stress? Once again, we
need to return to the anatomy of the nervous system to understand
the conscious control of stress. The medulla of the brain, just above
your neck, is the site where most of your autonomic functions are
controlled without conscious control.

This tiny area in the brainstem controls all of the major functions, such as heart rate, breathing, eye movements and hearing.

In this tiny area, all the major control centres are adjacent to one another. The importance of this proximity becomes apparent when you consider that, by controlling one area *consciously* (breathing), you can bring others under conscious control to a significant degree. In other words, because breathing is the only area that is under *both* conscious and unconscious control, you can control the heart rate by proxy, as it were, by consciously controlling the breathing. This forms the basis of most meditation techniques, which are known to control emotions and not only reduce heart rate but also to stabilise the *rhythm* of the heart, an uneven rhythm being the basis of many heart attacks.

Not only can we control the heart rate in this way, but we can also exert a significant control over emotions via the conscious control of breathing. The association between the *unconscious* control of emotions and breathing is easily demonstrated:

- when arguing, we take short breaths

- when we're worried, breathing becomes shallow

- when we're frightened, breath can actually become completely arrested

- when we're angry, our breathing becomes irregular

- surprise can cause a marked breathing imbalance in favour of inhalation rather than exhalation

Emotions are no more than an external manifestation of stress, so obviously emotions and stress – and breathing – are inextricably linked. But the only aspect that we can consciously control is the rate of breathing, and therefore concentrating on breathing permits control of emotions and control of stress.

And, because by controlling your breathing you are also controlling many other autonomic functions of the body that affect all of the other organs, it has a beneficial effect on several bodily processes.

How is breathing central to health?

To fully comprehend the central role of breathing in overall well-being, we obviously need to understand the various components of respiration. Breathing is divided into two separate areas:

- external respiration
- internal respiration

External respiration

External respiration is the physical act of breathing – oxygen passing across the membranes of the lungs into the bloodstream and carbon dioxide passing out of the body. Oxygen is required by every cell in the body to maintain life and vitality, and cellular death occurs very quickly if oxygen is not present. So even minor changes in lung function can have major effects on cellular health at a micro level, affecting general health at the macro level. And, as a direct corollary, this has major effects on the ageing process: as individual cells become sick and unable to function, ageing is accelerated.

Internal respiration

Internal respiration is the process occurring *within* the cells. The oxygen is transported by the red blood cells to the individual cells of the body and then is released into the cell. At this point the oxygen is required for reactions within the cell to produce energy from sugar (glucose), which is also supplied by the blood. As a by-product, carbon dioxide is released, which is toxic, and which needs to be removed from the body very quickly to prevent damage. This is transported in the blood to the lungs and expelled as we exhale.

Any interruption in the oxygen supply to the cells of more than a few minutes causes cellular death, ultimately leading to death, and therefore constant and careful control of breathing (without interruption) is absolutely essential.

Of course the importance of this is that the capacity of the lungs (known as the *vital capacity*) controls the amount of oxygen that we absorb. When we breathe normally at a relatively shallow rate of twelve to eighteen times per minute, we absorb about 7,500 cubic centimetres of air (of which 20 per cent is oxygen). By comparison, if we control breathing at approximately six breaths per minute with deep breaths involving the diaphragm, this increases to about 12,000 cubic centimetres per minute – almost twice as much oxygen absorption as the normal breathing rate with one-third of the breathing rate. This dramatically improves health by increasing the amount of oxygen available to the tissues, and, much more important, removing the toxic carbon dioxide from the body.

So, just by practising deep breathing through a meditative process, not only can we control our heart rate, reduce emotional instability and reduce stress, but we can also dramatically increase the recuperative powers of the body by increasing the amount of oxygen available and decreasing the amount of toxic carbon dioxide. On a macro level, consciously breathing rhythmically promotes smooth and even respiratory function, reduces the cycle of variation of the heart rate and brings about heart-rate stability; and, by stimulating autonomic functions and reducing stress, it causes a more stable function of the other major autonomic functions of digestion, immune regulation and the production of both red blood cells (to transport oxygen) and white blood cells (to fight infection).

And because the organs of the body and cellular functions are healthier, the process of ageing is inevitably slowed. Ageing occurs not only because of an increase in toxic substances in the cells (which is directly related to the amount of oxygen that we breathe and the carbon dioxide that we retain), but also as a direct result of the level of stress hormones, particularly if the stressful environment is unremitting. Deep, regular breathing balances the cardiorespiratory cycle – the close link between heart rate and breathing – through their anatomical association in the brainstem, thereby reducing stress levels, which slows the ageing process.

Control of the autonomic nervous system is very difficult but it can be achieved. In fact, it *must* be achieved if stress reduction is to be successful. And, as stress is a common predisposing factor in many of the serious physical illnesses that develop in men, the reduction of stress should be an absolute priority. As we have seen, it involves only a maximum of ten minutes per day – two five-minute periods – to achieve immensely successful results in terms of prevention of disease. Think of the exercise of the mind as being as important as the exercise of the body and you *will* find that ten-minute period per day.

The following examples describe cases where lifestyle changes have caused major health improvements. They also clearly demonstrate how health involves a combination of nutritional adjustment, stress control and exercise; they are all complementary and insufficient in isolation. The reduction of cortisol levels by appropriate diet and exercise is just as important as the de-stressing techniques described.

CASE HISTORY • ANDREW

Andrew is a forty-six-year-old corporate lawyer whose hectic lifestyle was driving him to a diagnosis of diabetes – rapidly. At 5 feet 9 inches (1.75m) and 107kg, he was grossly overweight, with poor concentration levels, lack of muscle tone and a blood pressure not to be envied. His initial blood tests revealed an elevated fasting blood glucose of 9.1 mmol/l (normal 5.8), so he was well on the way to developing diabetes. His insulin level (a predictive factor for diabetes) was 16.5 when the normal should be 5. Heart disease was also looming high on the agenda with a blood cholesterol of 6.8 mmol/l (normal 4).

→

Working eighteen-hour days under high stress, and the associated obligatory dinners and lunches and excessive alcohol intake, was taking its toll on his health. He was on a downward spiral with no obvious way out. As a corporate lawyer, in aggressive, confrontational situations on a regular basis, and concerned to be competing with younger, healthier men, he needed to address his health issues quickly.

Andrew embarked on an immediate change in his nutritional intake, commenced a light exercise regime and set aside specific times during the day to de-stress. Within two weeks he had lost 3kg and had noticeably more energy. After one month of lifestyle adjustment, his blood glucose had reduced to 6.4 (almost normal) and his insulin had reduced to 5.7 (from 16.5), almost completely eliminating his risks of diabetes. The cholesterol had been reduced to 5.2 mmol/l – so his risk of heart disease was much less – and he had reduced in weight by a massive 10kg, once again alleviating the strain on the heart that obesity causes.

Although he had a high-powered and intensely stressful job, he could make the necessary changes relatively easily and reverse the trend.

CASE HISTORY • DAVID

David is a forty-one-year-old banker under constant stress, who travels extensively both by air and rail. His lifestyle was controlled by the food available while travelling, which caused chronic indigestion from fast-food consumption. He was relatively fit, running for one hour on at least four days per week, but was finding it much more difficult as time progressed. Weighing in at 102kg with a height of 5 feet 11 inches (1.8m) was rather excessive, and his insulin measurement of 9.4 was almost double the normal (5 mIU/l). His cholesterol measurements were elevated at 5.8 and he was borderline diabetic at 6.1 mmol/l (normal 5.8).

Exercise was not an issue, because he was already factoring that into his lifestyle. The problem in his case was diet and stress. He had read extensively on nutrition issues and assumed he was following the best advice by stocking up on carbohydrates, especially before exercise. In fact, when we examined the issue, he was consuming the equivalent of up to 50 teaspoons of sugar per day as 'hidden' carbs in wraps, bagels, brown rice and pasta.

By planning healthy meals – restricting refined carbs and replacing them with more protein and vegetables, which was easily achieved despite his hectic lifestyle – within two weeks he was exercising with much more energy. He scheduled stress-releasing exercises twice per day specifically into his diary and ensured he never missed a session. Two weeks later, he had reduced in weight by 6kg, his insulin level had returned to almost normal at 5.2, his blood sugar level had returned to normal at 5.5 mmol/l and his cholesterol was 5.1, so he was heading for a healthy heart.

By planning the best choices of food on the move and incorporating stress-relief exercises into his daily regime, he was en route to weight reduction and reduced risk of heart disease – and he was running much faster.

CHILL OUT | 63

SUMMARY

▶ Stress is the reaction that controls virtually every action of your body.

▶ It is controlled by a dedicated nervous system – the autonomic nervous system – and by hormones such as cortisol.

▶ Stress is a causal factor in many medical problems such as obesity, myocardial infarction (heart attack), high cholesterol, diabetes, hypertension, strokes, stomach ulcers, back pain, reduced immunity and low libido.

▶ A major component of stress relates to our methods of coping with past experiences.

▶ Effective de-stressing requires developing voluntary control mechanisms for the autonomic nervous system – a unique concept for most individuals but achievable with practise.

▶ Controlling the stress reaction by natural methods is the only successful way to de-stress, so take control by not smoking, by establishing good eating habits and by following a good sleep regime.

▶ Controlled breathing is very effective because it is the only autonomic process that is also controllable at a conscious level, and by controlling breathing you can have an indirect effect on other systems such as heart rate.

CHAPTER 4

Are You Facing a Fat Dilemma?

The concept of 'fat' probably occupies more time in the psyche of people over forty than virtually any other topic. While your interest in active sport and amorous contemplation of others diminishes, abdominal fat just seems to keep on increasing, no matter what you do. And you can't get away from it. It is there when you dress in the morning, when you shower, and each time you look at a meal and think that perhaps you shouldn't be eating all of this.

However, most of the popular conceptions about body fat are actually 'misconceptions'. In fact, men have a greater level of misunderstanding about body fat than any other health-and-fitness topic.

The commonest misconceptions about body fat

You can burn up body fat by exercise

No, you can't. Body fat is controlled by certain hormones. Exercise elevates the level of the hormones that affect fat metabolism. You need to exercise for very long periods and also consume virtually no food to successfully burn up body fat by exercise – which is virtually impossible for most men.

The amount of fat around your abdomen is related to the number of calories you consume

Wrong again. Fat around the abdomen is deposited as a direct consequence of the hormone insulin (see Chapter 1). If you have low insulin levels, you can consume many more calories and still not deposit fat. As a direct corollary, if you have high insulin levels, fat will be deposited around the abdomen – even if you consume fewer calories. And, as we have already seen, insulin is stimulated by refined carbohydrates and stress. So abdominal fat is related to the *type* of food you eat rather than the *calorie content*.

Gradually increasing body fat is just an indicator of excessive eating

Still wrong, and for the same reasons as above. Increasing body fat is related to insulin, irrespective of the amount of food you consume.

You develop more fat cells as you get older

Actually, no. The number of fat cells when you are a teenager is the same number as you grow older – they just enlarge. Well, this is not *entirely* true. It's certainly the 'normal' response of fat cells to ageing but there are two major exceptions associated with modern lifestyles: liposuction can cause the body to replicate fat cells, and so can excessive overeating. More on that later.

Exercising one area of the body (for example, abdominal muscles) removes the fat from that area

Another common misconception. Fat deposition is controlled centrally, not locally, so exercising the abdominal muscles has no local action on fat removal.

Increased body fat is inevitable as you age

Just because most men become fatter with age, it does not mean that ageing is the cause. Fat is not a function of age: it is a function of lifestyle. You can adopt a healthy lifestyle as you age, which will prevent fat developing.

You don't need fat cells for health

Yes, you do. Body fat is absolutely essential to maintain a healthy body. Fat cells around the internal organs prevent damage. The problem arises when we develop too much.

All fat is bad

The final mistake. As we saw above, body fat is essential for various physical reasons, but the less obvious fats in the body are also essential. Fats in the blood carry food to the various organs and tissues; fats around the nerves allow them to function; and there are several fat-soluble vitamins (such as vitamins A, D, E and K). These vitamins are required for many essential purposes: vitamin A for eyesight, vitamin D for the structure of bones and teeth, vitamin E for its antioxidant properties in removing dangerous free radicals, and vitamin K for blood clotting, to name but a few of their many functions. (We'll learn more about free radicals and antioxidants in Chapter 10.) Without fat in your diet, you cannot absorb these essential vitamins, with serious and inevitable consequences for your health.

Rather than looking at the popular misconceptions of fat, the most sensible approach would be to look at what fat cells are, how they develop and, much more importantly, how we can make them reduce in size, because an important point to realise is that, although, on occasions, fat cells can increase in number, they never actually go away. You can reduce them to a very small size but not make them disappear completely.

What is fat?

Basically, fat occurs in many different parts of the body, not just the abdomen. We have:

- Structural fat. This includes the fat that is part of the cell membrane and all the 50 trillion cells in the body.

- Blood fat. This is the fat travelling in the bloodstream to provide energy (triglycerides) and either to protect against heart disease (HDL) or to cause heart disease if in excess (LDL, triglycerides).

- Hormonal fat. The fats in your hormones are chemical messengers in your body.

- Fats around the nerve sheaths. These fats allow the nerves to function effectively.

- Storage fat. This fat occurs in two forms:

  - White fat: This is the commonest type of fat and makes up most of what you would normally consider to be fat: the fat around your waist and abdomen, which is actually storage of energy, and of which we are all aware.

  - Brown fat: Brown fat cells that are very specialised are situated, for instance, around your shoulder blades. These have particularly specialised roles in controlling body temperature under certain circumstances.

So it is immediately apparent that not all fat is bad. In fact, most of the fat in your body serves a very important purpose. There are other important reasons why body fat is so important.

- It acts as insulation. Subcutaneous fat (fat under the skin) protects us from loss of heat in the body (brown fat is actually a form of endocrine tissue, with specific metabolic capabilities, unlike the 'inert' white fat). Obviously, we don't need too much of this but a certain amount is important.

■ We need visceral fat. This is the fat that is situated around the organs and protects them. Once again, it is absolutely essential but when we have too much then it protrudes out into the belly (and is dangerous).

In this chapter, we are going to be concerned with two main forms of fat, which are the types that have particular effects, both negative and positive, on health:

■ white adipose tissue, the storage form of fat, mainly positioned in the abdomen, which we need to reduce to safe levels

■ the fats in the blood, which can either cause or protect against heart disease

Fortunately, both of these can be controlled relatively simply and efficiently by lifestyle changes, which are not difficult and are extremely effective.

But, if you really want to take control of body fat, it is essential to understand just exactly what fat cells are and what they look like. Around the abdomen in a man (hips and thighs in a woman) we accumulate fat cells – no surprise there.

Fat cells actually develop before birth, and merely tend to swell up during life, so, as we saw at the beginning of the chapter, the number of fat cells that you have at puberty tends to be, *in the majority of cases*, the same number you have later in life (although having liposuction, as we saw, can cause replication of fat cells, as can excessive eating). So, in the main, these cells tend to swell during life, and the development of a paunch is simply an accumulation of fat in single cells.

You can see, then, that fat cells (which have the medical term *adipocytes*) are simply like a swelling bag of fat. The fat that they include, of course, has the much more technical term of *triglyceride*; however, it is fat just the same.

But this mechanism of fat accumulation assumes a 'normal' diet and a 'normal' appetite. It was previously thought that the number

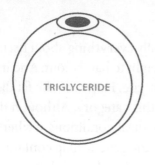
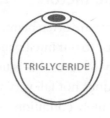

CONTAINING MORE FAT   CONTAINING LESS FAT

FAT CELLS

of fat cells that we were born with was the number we retained throughout life. However, *excessive overeating can undoubtedly increase the number of fat cells* and exacerbate the problem. So not only do you have fat cells that are enlarging in size, but also fat cells that can increase in number. The problem is that, if you do increase the number of fat cells by overeating, they will never disappear and you have them for the rest of your life.

The good news is that, although they won't disappear, you can actually shrink them to such a size that they are of little consequence. It is all simply down to lifestyle.

Distribution of body fat

Fat distribution is different in the sexes. Everyone knows that men have the typical upper-body, or 'apple', distribution, which is known as *android*. Women have the typical *gynoid* distribution in the lower body, which characteristically affects the hips and thighs and is pear-shaped.

But what determines this particular type of distribution? There are obviously several factors, some less important than others, so let's have a look at the ways in which this develops – and therefore how we can change it.

Genetic factors

Our genes are often blamed for virtually everything about us, from our shape to our intelligence, from weight to hair colour. And in the majority of cases this is undoubtedly true. However, the fat distribution does not fall very well under this category. Although there are definitely conditions – serious medical conditions – where fat distribution is determined directly by the genetic map contained in each of the cells of the body, in the majority of conditions genetics does not play a major role in the accumulation of excess fat. So I am afraid it is not an excuse for most of us.

Type of food intake

Surely this is obvious. If you consume the wrong types of food and too much of it then unfortunately you are probably going to be fat. But it is not quite as simple as that, which is why most weight-reducing diets are unsuccessful in changing body shape. If, for example, you go on a strict calorie-controlled diet, typically what happens is that you lose weight from the face and chest first and the last place that weight is lost from is the lump in the abdomen. There is a very serious medical reason for that.

Abdominal obesity, which is the type commonly known as the 'android' or 'apple' shape, is primarily caused by the hormone insulin. Insulin, as you saw in Chapter 1, is the hormone that actually deposits fat around your waist and in the visceral areas (around the organs), and causes so much damage to health. As we saw, the control of insulin is regulated primarily by restricting carbohydrate intake, specifically the high-GI foods such as bread, pasta and rice, which stimulate insulin very quickly and cause the production of fat. So, if you can reduce those foods, abdominal fat will start to disappear. And in this instance the abdominal fat will be the first to disappear, because, as insulin is responsible for depositing fat around the waist, *reducing* insulin will get rid of *that* fat first.

The simple expedient of reducing your high-GI food intake will automatically reduce insulin levels and start to burn fat from the abdomen, irrespective of the number of calories you eat. So, by merely changing the type of food you eat, you will alter your body shape automatically. It is inevitable. Physiologically, there is no way that this can be prevented.

So, is insulin the key to changing body shape and improving health? It is not quite as simple as that. There are several other factors affecting insulin as well as just diet, of which the most important is...

Stress

As we saw in Chapter 3, stress plays a very important part in health and weight. If you are highly stressed, for physical, emotional or psychological reasons, the effect is the same on the body: you produce more of a hormone called *cortisol*, and the cortisol works against insulin causing it to rise due to *insulin resistance*.

So, if you are stressed, your cortisol levels increase, insulin increases, and you deposit fat around the abdomen (and, more importantly, stop breaking down the fat around the abdomen).

But it gets worse. Fat cells (the *adipocytes*) actually have cortisol receptors, as all cells do, which cause the effects of cortisol to be exaggerated and enhanced, preventing further fat breakdown. So the net effect is that, if you have high levels of stress, your insulin levels are elevated, and you simply cannot either break down your own fat cells to release the energy stored within, or prevent food being converted into fat automatically.

Obviously, excess fat distribution around the waist is unsightly and unpleasant, but there are much more important health reasons for preventing this. Excess abdominal fat is associated with:

- increased risk of cardiovascular disease such as heart attack

- hypertension

- arthritis

- diabetes

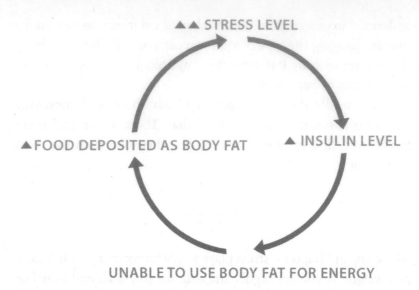

▲▲ STRESS LEVEL

▲ INSULIN LEVEL

▲ FOOD DEPOSITED AS BODY FAT

UNABLE TO USE BODY FAT FOR ENERGY

But of even more importance is visceral fat, which is associated with a greater risk of these conditions. The easiest way to check this is to measure your waist-to-hip ratio by measuring the circumference of your waist and dividing it by the circumference of your hips. If this is greater than 0.95, then problems are developing. Simply having a waist measurement greater than 40 inches poses an increased risk for medical problems from fat cells.

SUMMARY

▸ Fat in the body has many important functions. However, we are particularly concerned to remove the unsightly and dangerous fat cells around the abdomen.

▸ Most of the fat cells in your body were there at birth, and have merely expanded by accumulating more fat as time goes on.

→

▶ Fat cells around the abdomen are mainly controlled by the hormone insulin.

▶ Insulin is largely controlled by the intake of refined carbohydrates, especially high-GI foods such as bread, pasta, rice, cakes and confectionary.

▶ You can change body shape and improve your health by simply reducing these high-GI foods in your diet.

▶ Stress causes the production of the hormone cortisol, which increases the size of fat cells by acting against insulin. Therefore it is essential to reduce stress by following the techniques explained in Chapter 3.

▶ Although fat around the abdomen is unsightly, it is also an important marker of serious disease and increased risk of heart disease, hypertension, arthritis and diabetes.

▶ A waist-to-hip ratio of greater than 0.95 or a waist size greater than 40 inches is a significant risk factor.

▶ Exercising, though important for other reasons, does not reduce fat around the abdomen.

CHAPTER 5

The Importance of Fluid Balance

Water is the most important nutrient and component in your diet (and without doubt the least highly regarded). Incredible as it may sound, water actually makes up about 72 per cent of your body weight (excluding fat), which reduces to about 56 per cent as you age. So the 'average' man of 70kg consists of 45 litres of pure water.

Obviously, most of the water is contained in the 50 trillion (50,000,000,000,000) cells in the body, although a certain amount remains outside the cells and facilitates many of the body processes. And all of the myriad processes that occur in all of the cells of the body are entirely dependent on the hydration factor. In other words, the amount of water in your body determines virtually every process that will occur, and that is certainly a very sobering thought (even without alcohol!).

More importantly, this process is subject to very strict controlling factors. The loss of as little as 1–2 per cent of the fluid levels in the body results in significant dehydration, with all its attendant symptoms:

- headaches
- constipation
- dry mouth
- poor concentration
- irritability and low mood
- fatigue
- light-headedness
- dark-coloured urine, which can lead to kidney stones and pain
- poor vision
- increased joint pains

So it can be easily appreciated that even small changes in water content lead to immense problems for the body. A reduction in water content of only 10 per cent leads to cessation of all bodily functions.

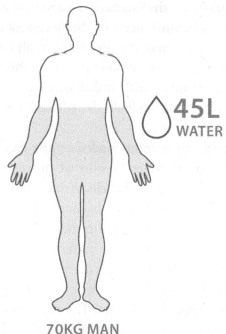

45L
WATER

70KG MAN

The problem is that the thirst mechanism is relatively inefficient. By the time you become thirsty you will have already lost
1–2 per cent of the fluid volume of the body and therefore you
will experience these symptoms at a very late stage in the process.
Most of the symptoms are relatively silent.

For example, when you become constipated, develop headaches
or become irritable, you don't immediately consider that your
body's water level is reducing and you are becoming dehydrated.
On the contrary, you might usually take some form of medication
for these symptoms, such as laxatives for constipation or aspirin
for headaches. We are beginning to treat the *effects* of the condition,
rather than the causes, and the causes are relatively simply treated
– just by drinking more water.

The problem with dehydration is that it is much commoner in
everyday life than you think. Everyone understands that, if you are
in a hot dusty climate, drinking lots of fluid is necessary to prevent dehydration. However, what few people realise is that the
atmosphere in the average office controlled by air conditioning is
actually drier than the Sahara desert and that water loss is increased
under these circumstances. The body cannot distinguish between
a very hot atmosphere and very extreme air conditioning in terms
of its water loss. You wouldn't normally think that, if you're in a
self-contained office with sealed windows and air conditioning,
you would become gradually dehydrated. But that is exactly what
happens.

This problem is compounded by the fact that our bodies are
constantly losing water by normal processes. Not only do we
require water in each of the cells to make those processes function
(of which more later) but we also need to lose a significant amount
of water per day to keep the body healthy.

About 50 per cent of the water loss per day is through the
kidneys in the urine, and this is essential to remove the waste products from the body. But less obvious is the fact that about 47 per
cent is lost through your skin. The more sweat you produce, the
more water you lose, but even in normal, everyday situations you

are losing a considerable amount of fluid. And, just to complete the picture, a small amount of water is lost in bowel motions, and – although less – through breathing.

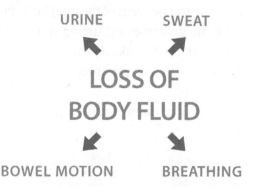

So you can see that, even if you are (apparently) doing nothing, you are losing water all the time. And this needs to be replenished – all the time. So how much water do we actually lose every day, without taking exercise or temperature into account? The average man aged 45–55 will lose about 2.5 litres per day without additional factors such as exertion taken into account. That is the equivalent of ten glasses of water. This figure obviously rises exponentially when exercise or external air temperature is included in the equation.

But the problem is not just water. Every time we lose water, we also lose essential electrolytes – such as sodium, potassium and calcium – which are essential for health and are also needed to control the fluid balance in the body. So, if you merely replace the water, you can become ill because you become electrolyte-depleted. This does not mean that you have to drink electrolyte-rich drinks marketed specifically for this purpose, but it does mean that you have to maintain a healthy, nutritionally balanced diet to ensure that all of these essential minerals are available, to prevent damage to the body. And it is the potential for damage to the body that we are discussing.

To examine this seriously, let us focus on the reactions occurring in a single cell rather than the whole body. It's relatively easy to tell when we're becoming dehydrated or constipated or irritable or fatigued, but these are very extreme symptoms after extreme fluid loss, as mentioned, of up to 2 per cent of the total body fluids. Much more important are the processes occurring in every individual cell, because the individual cells make up the body and, when they begin to become sick (and die), major processes that we recognise as diseases develop rapidly.

Cells in the body have the following appearance:

CELL MEMBRANE

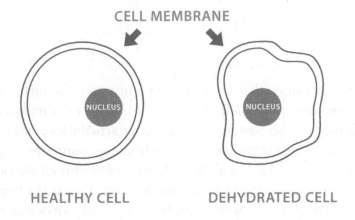

HEALTHY CELL   DEHYDRATED CELL

As you can see, there is a central nucleus, with a cellophane-like membrane enclosing something resembling a bag of water. Within that bag of water, the nucleus controls the processes and all the other materials (known as *organelles*), which convert the energy into action and make the body function. Of course, the cells are developed into different shapes and functions depending on the organ involved, so heart cells have a different shape from nerve cells or from liver cells, but the basic principles are the same for every cell in the body: each requires sufficient materials such as nutrients, energy and water to survive. If any one of these essential materials becomes depleted, damage occurs to the cell and, by definition, as the cells become more damaged, the body ages and diseases occur.

This really is the basis of ageing: quite simply, individual cell damage and death gradually accumulating into major diseases. By the time symptoms develop and are experienced, the damage is quite severe. Obviously, we are not suggesting that you can prevent ageing or even that you can prevent all diseases, but you can certainly prevent the progressive development of most diseases by maintaining nutrition and hydration. This would seem an incredible assertion to make. However, it is rather self-evident when you consider the matter. If the cell's basic requirements for water, electrolytes (such as sodium and potassium) and obviously energy sources (such as glucose) are not met, the cell becomes ill and ceases to function.

The combination of nonfunctioning and dead cells can lead to major diseases. And this is before we take into account the further complications resulting from major toxins such as alcohol and nicotine, affecting the liver and lungs.

Recognise the signs

Before you can combat the effects of ageing, you need to recognise the major signs. Some are obvious but some are certainly not so. Let us look at a few in turn.

Fatigue, both mental and physical

The brain is undoubtedly the organ in your body that is most susceptible to dehydration. Even mild variations in fluid levels in brain cells cause significant fatigue, low mood, irritability and lack of concentration. We are sure you will have recognised these symptoms at some point during your day, usually mid-afternoon, but perhaps you don't realise that the simple cause was dehydration. As we shall see later, coffee is definitely not the solution.

Physical fatigue is a little easier to explain. Obviously the muscles need to be hydrated and robust enough to fulfil the various functions of movement, but, much more importantly, the loss of electrolytes through dehydration (such as sodium and potassium) can exacerbate problems significantly.

Heart disease

The extreme effect that dehydration has on the heart is not usually recognised. Dehydration causes the stress reaction to be stimulated, and, as explained in Chapter 3, this has very significant effects on the constriction of arteries supplying the essential oxygen and nutrition to the heart muscle and increasing heart rate, both of which can lead to damage to the heart.

When your body-fluid level reduces, the amount of cholesterol in the blood increases. This is a very simple equation, since, if your fluid level reduces by 50 per cent (which is obviously a gross exaggeration for demonstration purposes), the concentration of blood cells and cholesterol will double. And, as cholesterol has the effect of increasing the viscosity of the blood, creating a 'sludging' effect, the blood will become more viscous and much more liable to block the arteries, causing potential heart disease.

Kidney disease

The kidneys remove most of the toxins from the blood, and therefore from the body, but they need lubrication to do this. And the lubrication is water. As we have seen, we tend to lose about 2.5 litres of water from our body per day, at least 1.25 litres via the kidneys. If we don't remove enough toxins, not only kidney disease but generalised illness occurs. So, by the simple expedient of drinking more water, you not only protect your kidneys but you protect all of the organs of the body. It is fairly easy to tell whether you are drinking enough water: simply look at the colour of your urine. If it is dark (at any time but first thing in the morning), because the toxins are too concentrated, you are simply not drinking enough water.

Constipation

Constipation is an increasing problem as we grow older, but it need not be so. Basically, the way in which our bowel functions is relatively simple: the muscle of the bowel responds to stretching, and if it is stretched it stimulates the bowel to push the matter down and out. And, as you know, the most effective material to 'stretch' the bowel is fibre, because fibre is made up of cellulose, which cannot be digested, so it just has to pass through. Fibre is most commonly present in fruit and vegetables and unrefined grains.

But the most important factor in preventing constipation is actually an adequate fluid intake. If the fibre does not have the lubrication that water provides, it doesn't move and constipation becomes inevitable.

Irritable bowel syndrome

Another important disease that can be significantly alleviated by adequate fluid intake is irritable bowel syndrome (IBS). This is commonly ascribed to stress, and stress is undoubtedly a major factor. However, what is generally less understood is that the irritable bowel is usually secondary to the overgrowth of an organism called candida. Candida lives in our bowel naturally but its weakness is that it can survive only on carbohydrates (sugars). When candida overgrows, usually due to a diet based on refined carbohydrates, it stimulates the bowel excessively and causes irritability and diarrhoea. Cut out the carbs, eradicate the candida, and much of IBS will disappear.

So drink plenty of water, be kind to your bowel, and prevent inflammatory diseases and even bowel cancer to a major degree.

Dehydration during exercise

Exercise is obviously very healthy (provided it is not taken to extremes). However, the potential effects of dehydration on joints and muscles are not usually fully understood.

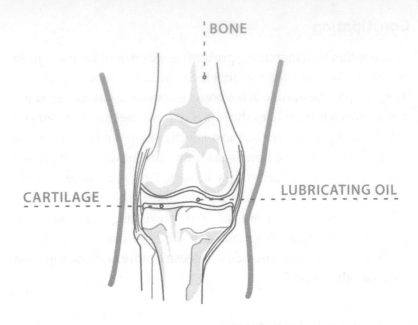

NORMAL JOINT

Basically, most joints have two bony surfaces separated by an oily fluid that allows lubrication. The bone surfaces are covered by cartilage, and the bones should really never come into contact with one another, otherwise it can be painful. The oil lubricates the joints and prevents this from happening. When we exercise we obviously place much more stress on the joints, particularly the hip, knee and joints of the ankle, which take a severe beating each time you run. However, they are built for that, provided you prepare correctly. Everyone knows that you need energy during exercise, and therefore taking in appropriate energy beforehand is an accepted fact. But not everyone realises the importance of hydration in exercise. Although it is not instantly apparent, there is fluid within the cartilage and obviously between the parts of the joint. When you exercise, dehydration increases and it is important to ensure sufficient fluid intake to replace the water that has been lost. If you don't replace the fluid, the body has to take emergency measures, one of which is to protect the brain. As a final stage of dehydration, fluid is lost from brain cells, and the tissues of the body take protective measures to prevent that occurring. Therefore fluid is taken from other tissues in preference, and among the least important, unfortunately, are the joints. So fluid is lost from the joints in preference during exercise and this causes the surfaces to come closer together, creating the potential for pain and arthritis. By the simple expedient of sufficient fluid intake before, during and after exercise, you can prevent this happening to a major degree.

Similarly, the muscles are subject to dehydration during exercise. Exercise causes the loss of a considerable volume of fluid because body temperature rises and external temperatures increase. When you exercise to extreme levels, muscles are unable to obtain sufficient oxygen for normal usage (aerobic) and therefore they develop a method of contracting without oxygen (anaerobic), but this causes the build-up of a substance called *lactic acid*, which causes pain.

We are sure most runners have experienced extreme pain in the calves when running perhaps a little more than they should, and this is the cause. You need water to wash the lactic acid out.

How to solve the problem of dehydration

The simple answer is to drink more water, but how much? Obviously, the fluid intake required depends on the activity involved, the external circumstances (such as temperature) and individual lifestyle. There are, however, several basic rules that you need to follow to prevent dehydration and therefore prevent these conditions developing. As a general rule, the minimum amount of fluid (as water) intake per day is half your body weight (measured in pounds) in fluid ounces. So an average 160-pound person would require 80 fluid ounces (4 British pints or 2.27 litres) of water per day, which is about 10 cups. And this is pure water, not including other fluids such as tea or coffee. In fact, it is important to bear in mind that some fluids will contribute to dehydration. Here are a few of them.

- Alcohol. We don't want to seem like total killjoys on alcohol, because in moderation there is no problem, but excess alcohol definitely causes significant dehydration and all the conditions described above.

- Sugar-filled drinks. These are high in carbohydrates (sugars). Carbohydrates store water and therefore they can cause a form of 'internal dehydration' by locking up the water. In addition, every molecule of sugar needs a molecule of water to break it down into two molecules of glucose (a simple sugar), meaning a requirement for more water. So excessive refined carbohydrates in any form contribute to dehydration.

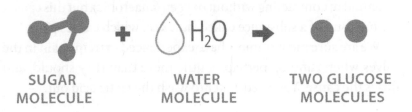

| SUGAR | WATER | TWO GLUCOSE |
| MOLECULE | MOLECULE | MOLECULES |

- Caffeine: Caffeine causes dehydration. You have to restrict your coffee intake both to reduce insulin levels and to reduce the requirement for water, or drink more water. Interestingly, the caffeine in tea seems to have a lesser effect, which may be due to the healthy antioxidants in tea.

In general, it is safest to drink too much water than too little. The golden rule is: never wait until you are thirsty before replenishing the body-fluid levels. As we have seen, thirst occurs at a late stage (approximately 1–2 per cent dehydration) and at this stage damage is definitely occurring to the cells. Consume the minimum amount of water above (at least 10 cups per day) in addition to your normal tea, coffee or soft-drink intake (which will obviously be low because of the added sugar).

How does exercise affect this equation? As a general rule, about 500ml (almost a UK pint) of water should be consumed every two hours for the twenty-four hours prior to extreme exercise, and about 200ml (0.35 pint) every twenty minutes during extreme exercise. But remember that during extreme exercise pure water can be slightly dangerous. Strenuous exercise (such as marathons or sports involving hours of continuous exertion) will result in electrolytes (such as sodium and potassium) being lost, so you need to replace the fluids under these circumstances with water *plus electrolyte additions* to avoid significant mineral deficiencies.

What *can* you drink?

Well, water obviously. It is probably best to have water immediately available at your work station and to drink at least ten cups per day. During strenuous exercise, drinking water with electrolyte additions, which is widely available in shops and supermarkets, is by far the safest.

Fruit juice is far too high in sugar for general consumption, so add a little fruit juice to a quantity of water for safety. Vegetable juices, on the other hand, are much safer and much lower in sugar and have much higher levels of nutrition.

As we have seen, caffeine produces dehydration (and also cardiac arrhythmias), so take a maximum of two coffees per day. Tea is a little less stimulating so you could have three cups. Herbal tea is an excellent alternative. There are many herbal teas, which have effects from relaxation to stimulation, and all are extremely healthy with virtually no health restrictions.

Alcohol can be taken, but in moderation, and definitely not more than two small glasses of wine per day.

Warning: be careful of 'healthy' sports drinks. Many sports drinks have lots of excellent additives such as the minerals we lose during exercise, but many also contain a lot of sugar, so always read the label.

Can you drink too much water?

The answer is 'yes', but it is almost impossible. Obviously, the problem is that if your intake of fluid is much more than your output, then you develop lower levels of sodium and this can cause severe problems. But to do this you need to drink more than about 8 litres per day, and that is virtually impossible under normal circumstances.

SUMMARY

▶ The effects of dehydration can lead to:

▸ diabetes

▸ stress

▸ kidney disease

▸ raised blood pressure

▸ headaches

▸ skin disorders

▸ constipation

▸ fatigue

▸ gall stones

▸ bowel disease

▸ palpitations

▸ arthritis

▸ mood swings

▶ Simply consume more fluid as pure water. How easy can it be?

6

Alcohol – the Facts

No book on men's health would be complete without a section on alcohol, primarily because alcohol plays such a major part in men's health, especially after the age of forty. But in order to deal with this safely and effectively, you really need to understand, first, exactly what alcohol is, and, second, how it can affect you. Before continuing, we should emphasise that we are not advocating an anti-alcohol approach, although it may appear so from the initial paragraphs, merely a medical approach to enjoying alcohol safely (if you wish to) and, more importantly, offering an explanation of the hidden effects of consuming alcohol to excess regularly.

Basically, alcohol is *ethanol* or *ethyl alcohol*, and is exactly the same whether in spirits, beer, cider or wine.

The only difference between these various alcoholic drinks is the amount of alcohol and the other ingredients in them (such as sugar) that affect the taste, and this depends on how the alcohol was produced (either by fermentation or distillation) in the first place. But the single most important fact is that alcohol is a *sedative*, not a *stimulant*.

Surely that must be wrong, you're thinking. Everyone knows

that, when you drink alcohol, you become less inhibited, initially happy, and certainly seem stimulated. What is actually happening is that *social* inhibitions are the first to be released, causing (initially) a lowering of the anxiety levels natural in social situations. You can converse with relative strangers without a problem, a situation often more difficult without the apparent stimulus of alcohol.

The problem is that alcohol depresses functions in the body at different rates, and can initially appear stimulatory when what is happening is depression of the parts of the brain affecting *judgement*. In other words, initially you are losing control of your inhibitions.

The major effect of alcohol is to depress the activity of the brain, but many other effects on different organs of the body occur after that.

As loss of inhibitory functions continues, cerebral control over drinking more alcohol becomes lost and eventually alcohol effectively takes over your functions. Everybody knows the signs of intoxication:

- slurred speech

- blurred vision

- markedly decreased reaction times

- memory loss

- fatigue

- eventually a lack of control over basic bodily functions

Now obviously this is the extreme scenario and most people would not reach this level, but the point is that – to the body – the effects of alcohol in lesser amounts is the same but merely to a lesser degree. Although you may not ever reach this stage of intoxication, the effects on all these bodily functions *are* occurring every time you imbibe. The reason why we have to look at alcohol very carefully is that it is probably the most significant cause of the ageing effect in men in their forties onwards, and in some cases from the twenties onwards. The unhealthy effects of alcohol on various organs – not only the liver – will be explained later in the chapter.

But how does alcohol cause such a rapid effect on cerebral function?

It is possible to feel the effects of alcohol within minutes of drinking and the reason is that alcohol is one of the few substances that is absorbed in the stomach, rather than just the intestine. About 80 per cent of alcohol is absorbed directly through the stomach lining and directly into the venous system passing round the body, the remaining 20 per cent being absorbed in the next part of the gut, which is the small intestine.

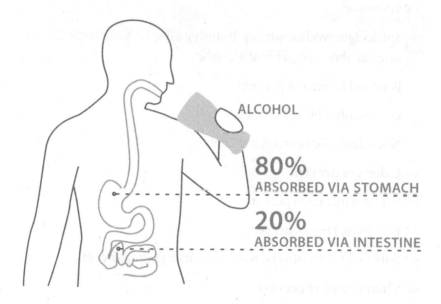

ALCOHOL

80%
ABSORBED VIA STOMACH

20%
ABSORBED VIA INTESTINE

So alcohol is absorbed within minutes of being consumed, particularly if on an empty stomach. When the alcohol enters the bloodstream, it is immediately passed to all the organs of the body, including the brain, the heart, the kidneys and the liver.

And, even worse, because alcohol is diluted in water in the body (it is how it passes through the system), organs (such as the brain) that have a high proportion of water and a rich blood supply (transporting the alcohol) are particularly susceptible to alcohol in the early stages of ingestion. Obviously, the more diluted the alcohol, the less its effect, which is why it is very important to drink as much water as possible if you intend to consume alcohol.

In this regard, it is important to stress the difference between men and women, because, as we all know, women can become intoxicated on less alcohol than men. There are many reasons for this, but one of the most important is that muscle tissue contains more water than fat tissue, and, as women tend to have a higher body fat index than men, obviously they have proportionally less water in the body and therefore the alcohol is less diluted and more effective. So how much alcohol is actually in the various drinks that we consume?

- Spirits (gin, vodka, whisky, brandy): all spirits are basically the same at about 40 per cent alcohol

- Beer and lager: 4–6 per cent

- Low-alcohol beer: 1.5 per cent

- Non-alcoholic beer: 0.5 per cent

- Cider 4–6 per cent

- White wine: 12–13 per cent

- Red wine: 12–14.5 per cent

- Fortified wines (sherry, port, Madeira): 18–21 per cent

- Champagne: 12 per cent

It would appear at a glance that wine is more alcoholic than beer, which, quantity for quantity, it is; but you have to consider the amount normally consumed in addition to the proportion of alcohol. It would be unusual to drink a pint of wine (hopefully), but not unusual to drink several pints of beer. A glass of wine is about 175ml and a pint of beer is 568ml, so you can see that, on those figures, there is obviously more alcohol in a pint of beer (approximately 3 x 5 per cent) than a standard glass of wine (13 per cent).

Of course, there is much more to alcohol that can cause medical problems than just the ethanol content. For example, beers, which have high carbohydrate content (sugars), have a greater likelihood of promoting the development of diabetes than those drinks with a low carbohydrate content, such as red wine.

So what happens to the alcohol once it passes through the stomach lining into the bloodstream?

Depending on the concentration of the alcohol consumed, it can actually start to cause organ damage the second you start drinking. Concentrated alcohol, such as neat spirits (or slightly diluted spirits) cause inflammation of the oesophagus (the tube leading to the stomach) and the lining of the stomach itself, which can become very inflamed, causing ulcers and bleeding.

And, of course, it is important to remember that, because alcohol passes across the stomach lining immediately into the bloodstream, which obviously travels to all the organs of the body, all of the organs are affected by alcohol within a question of minutes. So, for example, the kidneys, heart, brain and liver are all affected by the alcohol within minutes of ingestion. And the immediate effect of alcohol is to cause the blood vessels within all these organs to dilate, an effect that is fairly obvious on the skin when you become red and sweat after taking a little more alcohol than perhaps you should.

It is also worth noting that the colder the alcohol, the more slowly it is actually absorbed – an excellent reason for always having cold beer or ice in your drinks. This may account, in part, for why alcohol problems are so prevalent in Japan, where warm Saki is consumed in preference to cold Saki, although there are other medical reasons which are also responsible.

Let us sum up so far.

- All alcohol is basically a form of ethanol or ethyl alcohol.

- It is absorbed through the stomach wall and therefore has a rapid effect.

- After being absorbed into the bloodstream it passes to all the major organs, including the brain, and has immediate effects.

- Alcohol is a sedative, and never a stimulant.

- It appears to have initial stimulating effects, however this is as a result of it suppressing the inhibitory centres in the brain – ultimately it causes drowsiness.

- It has more rapid effects on women because of their higher fat-to-body weight ratio.

- The more dilute the alcohol, the slower the absorption.

- The colder the alcoholic beverage, the more slowly the alcohol is absorbed.

What is the 'blood alcohol level'?

Alcohol infiltrates the bloodstream, passes to the organs, and it is the concentration of alcohol in the bloodstream that determines its effects, which is known as the *blood alcohol level*. So, the blood alcohol level is, quite simply, the proportion of alcohol in the blood. There are several ways in which this can be affected.

As we have seen, the more dilute the alcohol, the slower the rate of absorption and the lower the blood alcohol. This would seem rather obvious, but several other effects of alcohol are not quite so obvious. The blood alcohol level increases when alcohol is consumed on an empty stomach. Once again, fairly obvious, as the alcohol can be absorbed more quickly without being mixed with other contents. However, not quite so obvious is the fact that the bubbles (the carbon dioxide) in carbonated mixers (such as cola and lemonade) actually increase the absorption of alcohol and accelerate the elevation of the blood alcohol level. So a spirit taken with a carbonated mixer will actually have a more rapid effect on inhibitory actions that a spirit with a noncarbonated mixer. Fruit juices, on the other hand, slow the absorption process.

How do we eliminate alcohol from the body?

Alcohol is metabolised (broken down) by the liver, and then the residual parts are passed out of the body (excreted) by the kidneys (as urine), the skin (sweat) and the lungs (breathing). Obviously, just exactly how intoxicated we become depends on the balance between the amount of alcohol consumed and the rate at which the alcohol can be metabolised.

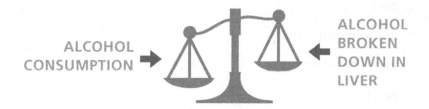

ALCOHOL CONSUMPTION → ← ALCOHOL BROKEN DOWN IN LIVER

THE INTOXICATION BALANCE

The rate of excretion (elimination) of alcohol is about 1 fluid ounce of alcohol per hour, or, in practical terms:

- 30ml of spirits

- 1 pint of beer

- 1 large glass of wine

So, if you have five large glasses of wine, it is going to take five hours for the alcohol to be eliminated from the system. As a typical bottle of wine is about five glasses, that is the equivalent of five hours per bottle.

What are the adverse effects of alcohol on the body?

Alcohol has undoubtedly some beneficial effects in moderation: it is well established that up to two glasses of red wine per day can have a preventive effect on the development of heart disease. However, alcohol in excess of this amount can have major deleterious effects on many organs of the body, not just the liver. To enlarge on this, we are going to look at a number of different anatomical regions of the body, as obviously alcohol has the capacity to affect them all:

- brain and nervous system

- liver

- gastrointestinal tract

- muscular system

- heart

- pancreas

- glandular system

- blood

The brain and nervous system

The brain and the nervous system show the most obvious signs of the effects of alcohol: its effects on the brain is why most people drink alcohol, as they seek 'relaxation' and lowered social inhibition. But the social-inhibition function is only the beginning of what may eventually become a very damaging effect on the body. The problem stems from the fact that different parts of the brain are affected by alcohol at different times. This means that, as the social-inhibition function is affected first, it seems to present an impression of stimulation. And social stimulation and the lowering of inhibition are pleasurable, so the motivation to drink more alcohol is self-evident. The problem is that, from that stage onwards, the effects of alcohol are all damaging, to both the brain and the rest of the body. Even worse, every time you drink too much, brain cells die and can never be recovered. The external signs of consuming excessive quantities of alcohol are obvious to everyone, but briefly occur in the following sequence.

- Reduced intellect with inability to make sensible judgements.

- Impairment in sensory and motor control with reduced sensation to pain and, obviously, lack of control of motor functions.

- Lack of control of the body's automatic mechanism, the autonomic nervous system, which controls functions such as the urinary tract, heart rate and breathing. The problem is compounded by the fact that, as the brain is the first organ to be affected (and obviously the most important), the lack of control is simply a vicious circle, which continues with further lack of control.

The effects of regular excessive consumption of alcohol are initially small but ultimately very serious:

- loss of memory

- confusion

- mood swings

- lack of control of behaviour

- loss of consciousness

- an early death

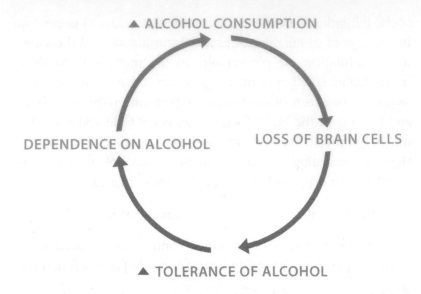

Alcohol reduces the amount of oxygen being transported to the brain, and every time you become intoxicated you lose thousands of the essential brain cells, which can never be recovered. Much worse than this is the fact that alcohol produces dependency on and tolerance to alcohol itself, whereby the vicious cycle continues.

The liver

Although the brain demonstrates most of the effects of alcohol externally, the liver bears the brunt of the problem. Cirrhosis of the liver is well recognised, but the problems reach much further. It is important to appreciate the actions of the liver, and the essential importance of the liver in your ultimate health, because it is the most important detoxifying organ in the body and if it is damaged the toxins will build up and cause serious medical problems. Almost all of the blood from the bowel is taken directly to the liver for processing and detoxifying, and therefore that is where alcohol is substantially broken down, or metabolised.

The essential functions of the liver that are disrupted by alcohol include:

■ removing toxins and poisons from the body

■ breaking down alcohol (yes – alcohol actually prevents its own metabolism by the liver, another vicious circle)

■ controlling the blood-fat levels in the body (such as cholesterol and triglycerides)

■ reducing antibodies to assist the immune system

■ producing bile that helps you digest foods

■ storing carbohydrates as glycogen

These are just a few of the many functions of the liver, and, while this is not intended to be a medical textbook, it is important to realise that if you damage the liver, even slightly, you damage all of these functions and your life expectancy will be reduced – even if you don't develop cirrhosis.

The gastrointestinal tract

The GI tract is the tube that runs from your mouth to your anus, and all that happens in between. So it includes:

■ the oesophagus

■ the stomach

■ the small intestine

■ the large intestine

■ associated organs such as the pancreas

And as we have already seen, alcohol can start to affect the GI tract from the moment of ingestion, causing inflammation of the oesophagus and increased acid in the stomach, leading to inflammation (indigestion) and ulcers. A peptic ulcer can rupture and lead to death. It also leads to capillary rupture. Capillaries

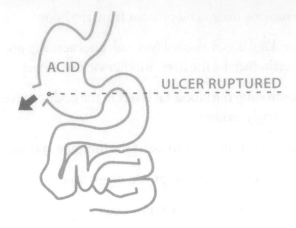

ACID

ULCER RUPTURED

EFFECT OF ALCOHOL ON THE STOMACH

are the small blood vessels all over the body, but they become obvious when you see blotches on facial skin and red eyes after a night of binge drinking.

The muscular system

Fatigue and tiredness after consuming alcohol are well recognised. However, what is not quite so obvious is that the reason is, once again, that the reduced blood flow to the muscles (as the blood vessels throughout the body are dilated) mean that they are just not receiving the oxygen they need for health, leading to a build-up of toxins.

The heart

Alcohol in excess can have very severe effects on the heart. The heart is a pump made of muscle, with an intrinsic nervous system that causes it to beat. If alcohol damages heart muscle, you can develop enlargement of the muscle, so it does not receive enough oxygen. This is called *cardiomyopathy*. You can also experience abnormality of the heart rate or irregular heartbeats (*arrhythmias*), which can lead to a myocardial infarction (heart attack).

The pancreas

The pancreas has many functions in producing secretions that help us to digest food, but its other important function is to produce the hormone insulin, which controls blood sugar. Excess alcohol intake causes blood-sugar levels to rise and the response of the pancreas is to produce more insulin, which then lowers the blood sugar.

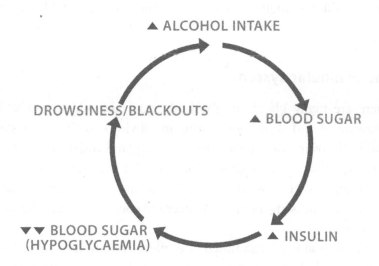

The problem is that, if your blood sugar reduces too quickly, you develop a low blood-sugar level (hypoglycaemia), and this causes drowsiness. The early symptoms include:

- poor concentration
- sweating
- anxiety
- low mood
- light-headedness

But, if it progresses to excess, loss of consciousness can occur. Even worse, if the pancreas is stimulated to produce too much

insulin for too long, it simply cannot keep functioning and diabetes results with its consequent side effects of:

- nerve damage

- kidney damage

- eyesight problems

It is not widely recognised that the commonest cause of blindness
in those between 18 and 65 is diabetes.

The glandular system

There are many glands in the body, some of which you will
be aware of and some not. Some are obvious, such as the sex
glands (the ovaries and testes), the thyroid gland and the pancreas.
Once again, as a sedative, alcohol reduces the function of these
glands and therefore we don't produce as much of the hormones
or chemical messengers the body needs to control certain essential
functions.

We have already examined the effects on the pancreas but
in men alcohol can have much more obvious effects on sexual
function. The problem is that it obviously affects the brain first of
all and causes a lowering of social inhibition, which *seems* in some
cases to be a sexual stimulant. But in fact alcohol is a sedative and
effectively has actions precipitating impotence, with:

- reduction in the erectile ability of the penis

- reduction in penis size during erection

- reduction in the size of the testes, with an increase in the female
  hormone oestrogen, causing female characteristics to develop,
  such as a change in pubic hair and the development of breasts
  ('man boobs', or 'moobs'); these are known as *secondary sexual
  characteristics* and are definitely to be avoided

Elevated blood alcohol levels can also:

- increase blood fats, causing heart disease, strokes and hypertension
- increase the risk of gout
- reduce immunity from infection
- reduce immunity, which can help the body fight cancer (it is well recognised that alcohol is associated with increased cancer rates)
- affect the bone marrow, which reduces our ability to make white blood cells and reduces our immunity to both cancers and infection

So you can see that excess alcohol consumption is definitely to be avoided, if you want to maintain a healthy lifestyle and a high standard of life for as long as possible.

SUMMARY

- ▶ It is the concentration of alcohol in the bloodstream that determines its effects.
- ▶ Elimination of alcohol from the system is at the rate of about 1 fluid ounce per hour.
- ▶ Alcohol has some beneficial effects: up to two glasses of red wine per day can have a preventive effect on the development of heart disease.
- ▶ However, excess alcohol consumption has the potential to affect every organ in the body, including the brain, the heart, the blood and the glandular system.
- ▶ Alcohol can also adversely affect the immune system, reducing your resistance to such illnesses as cancer.

CHAPTER 7

The Andropause (or 'Male Menopause') – Fact or Fiction?

Does the andropause – otherwise known as the male menopause – actually exist? In one sense, no, because *menopause* means the end of the monthly fertility cycle and, as men do not have one, by definition they cannot have a male menopause. But the andropause is a recognised series of symptoms and signs relating directly to the effects of reductions in testosterone levels that happen in most men from age forty onwards (or even earlier in some cases). Initially identified as a specific clinical entity in Australia, these symptoms can be wide-ranging, of varying strengths and are age-related.

What is the hard evidence?

Testosterone facts

- Testosterone levels fall as men get older.

- After the age of forty testosterone levels fall by about 1–2 per cent per year.

- By age seventy, 20 per cent of men are testosterone-deficient.

■ By age eighty, the level of testosterone in men is usually at pre-pubertal levels.

Learn to recognise the signs

Reduction in testosterone levels does *not* mean loss of reproductive ability. However, typical early-warning signs include:

■ fatigue, lack of energy

■ reduced libido

■ difficulty initiating and sustaining erections

■ increased irritability and mood swings

■ joint aches, especially affecting the hands

■ depression

All of the above can have other causes, a typical example being stress, but the difficulty here is a chicken-and-egg scenario: which came first?

Lowered testosterone can be caused by exposure to certain chemicals or pesticides found in particular work conditions. The majority of men, however, experience an almost unnoticeable decrease in testosterone levels as they grow older, and, as with so many facets of middle age, it is the insidious nature that makes it difficult to detect, because the symptoms and signs are so apparently unrelated. For example, sexual problems with potency and libido are an obvious corollary of the andropause, but depression, unexplained fatigue and mood swings are not so obvious.

The symptoms and signs of male depression secondary to the andropause are not commonly recognised in the early stages for many reasons:

■ Men have a denial response to illness, especially mental illness, and often refuse to accept its existence and therefore refuse to seek help.

- Men are often in a state of denial regarding sexual problems, too, considering these relate to a sense of perceived failure.

- The association between sexual problems and underlying depression is seldom made.

- Finally, and most importantly, the symptoms of male depression in midlife may be very different from the *typical* symptoms of depression.

Depression is greatly underdiagnosed in men. They tend to deal with low mood by persisting in their self-destructive lifestyle, at increasing cost to themselves physically, psychologically and socially. They battle on – but there are no medals for stoicism.

The majority of us do nothing to combat stress, opting simply to live with it. A poll shows that, while half of respondents said they felt stressed at least once a week and one in five every day, nearly two-thirds admitted they would not take any steps to deal with stress.

Unmanaged, stress can additionally develop into mental-health problems, as well as increasing the risk of physical problems. This highlights the problem of the unwillingness of men to accept that the body and the brain sometimes need repair. They acknowledge the expertise of garage and washing-machine mechanics but not that of doctors or, heaven forbid, psychologists.

They might see a physiotherapist – football clubs have physios, so it's OK. But consult a doctor or psychologist on their own daily performance? No way. Why the lack of logic?

The andropause male will often display the following behaviour:

- They will blame others for their own mistakes.

- They will display an overdeveloped fear of failure.

- They are frequently angry and irritable.

- They display massive mood swings.

- They show increased hostility.

These are not the typical signs of depression and so not the easiest to diagnose. More importantly, how do you treat this form of depression? Medication is not the answer in the majority of cases. Many antidepressants can actually cause impotence and sexual dysfunction, thereby exacerbating the problem.

While there is understandable controversy over the exact time when symptoms of andropause develop, this is usually when the testosterone level has dropped by about 50 per cent, although it can certainly occur prior to this stage. Replacement therapy with testosterone is reserved for severe cases (which will be discussed later in the chapter); in the majority of instances, there are very simple alternative approaches – primarily based on recognition of the specific problem – that assist in the alleviation of the low mood associated with the condition. So where might these problems lie?

Career and lifestyle issues

The 40–50 age range represents a changing lifestyle for many men. Success has either been achieved or not, as the case may be, but there is a gradual acceptance that future development is unlikely. This can lead to feelings of inadequacy or lack of success. Many different events are possible – even likely – at this time, including:

- separation/divorce
- children leaving home
- unemployment
- career displacement by a younger male
- illness, either to yourself or your partner

These are much more likely predisposing factors behind low mood or depression during the andropause than reduced testosterone levels; recognise the cause and deal with it for a successful resolution, as we will explain later in the chapter.

Acute testosterone deficiency

Acute, or sudden, reduction in testosterone levels is relatively rare. It results in a range of physical, sexual, emotional or psychological symptoms:

- Sexual problems are usually a weaker sex drive, difficulty in achieving and maintaining an erection and lowered sensitivity.

- Depression, irritability, poor concentration plus forgetfulness are the associated psychological symptoms.

- Physical signs include tiredness, muscle weakness, joint pain, dry skin and weight gain around the midriff.

When several of the symptoms are present concurrently at an early age (40–50), then a simple test of the testosterone level will reveal if medical treatment is required. Opinion is divided on the use of testosterone supplements. Unsupervised, unnecessary prescription of testosterone is at least unwise, if not positively dangerous to health.

Identify the real problem – then deal with it

Many of the symptoms listed above could be the outcome of other aspects of a less-than-positive lifestyle: employment pressures, poor eating patterns, unhelpful ways of handling the events of daily life. Adjust to the reality of the situation. The effects of this almost imperceptible reduction in vigour can be managed by using those very work skills you have probably practised over the years:

- identify the problem
- review the possible causes
- choose a remedy/solution
- test the chosen solution
- monitor the outcome

Sexual difficulties

Libido

All the usual problems of daily life – work overload, worry, stress – can lead to loss of sex drive and erectile function. Do not suffer in silence, as that may increase inner tensions. These in turn can reduce the likelihood of normal function. Treat this like any other physical change: obtain a specialist opinion and discover how you can turn the situation around. Take charge.

Poor diet and personal circumstances can affect libido. One survey found that most couples have sex more on a one-week holiday than during two months at home. More than half said they had sex ten times on holiday, yet 57 per cent made love only once a week at home. Which proves that sun, sea, sand and relaxation can be more effective than Viagra.

Poor nutrition causes physical and mental fatigue, leaving little left over for social interest, let alone sexual activity. Fatty diets have been found to lower sperm count. Obesity limits libido. In France obese men were 69 per cent less likely to have had more than one sexual partner in a year than men of normal weight.

Impotence

Impotence can also be an early sign of coronary artery disease and diabetes. Impotence can be due to atherosclerosis – a systemic condition where plaque builds up inside the arteries, leading to restricted blood flow in the penis.

This demonstrates why it's so important for men to talk to their doctor about impotence because it could be an early sign of heart and circulatory disease. If impotence is a problem, request a health check and a review of risk factors such as high blood pressure or diabetes.

Unfortunately many men are too embarrassed to discuss impotence with their doctors. Not only does such behaviour impact negatively on their quality of life, it also increases their risk of heart disease.

Physical changes

As we have seen, the physical signs of tiredness, muscle weakness and joint pain are usually the outcome of a demanding – and usually less-than-optimal – lifestyle. Poor nutrition and broken sleep patterns aggravate these signs. Tackle them simply and positively. Improve your diet. Reduce alcohol and coffee consumption. Reduce commitments where possible. Spend more time with family and friends in relaxing, noncompetitive (therefore stressfree) activities – and spend more time outdoors.

Dry skin and weight gain around the midriff are commonly accepted signs of approaching maturity – but this need not be the case. Moisturisers deal with the first. Many stores, companies and pharmacies have produced ranges of moisturisers aimed specifically at men. Women don't have a monopoly on skincare: your skin is simply a large body organ as worthy of attention and suitable products as your teeth and armpits. And don't forget to constantly replenish your fluid intake: dehydration is the commonest cause of dry skin and all of its associated complications (see Chapter 5 for more on the importance of hydration).

The weight gain round the middle requires more effort and attention but we have already solved this problem in Chapter 4.

Changing habits of eating and patterns of exercise hold the key to improvement. Exercise is known to be helpful in preventing and moderating depression. Add that to increased fitness and you get two benefits for the price of one.

Psychological challenges

Every business hits its difficult patches. Turnaround in business requires the ability of people to address problems, to break through the limits of their background and to change their usual habits. Adapting to change is always difficult – especially with increasing age – and can lead to psychological problems that can be ascribed to 'andropause', whereas they are natural stressful issues that cause the problems *associated* with the andropause. But adapting successfully, against the odds, can have the opposite effect: a sense of achievement, which elevates mood. By harnessing the power of motivation and resilience, which are *characteristics* of youth but are not *exclusive* to youth, you can overcome psychological problems.

As men, we often do what is required to improve a company but will not do the same for our own relationships, our own mental and physical health. Are our priorities all wrong?

There is one area of life at forty that can be a source of disappointment and requires adjustment. By forty most people have reached a plateau in their careers. Wherever that shining future may be, it is not in front of them. Letting go of a set of unfulfilled ambitions is never easy.

Now is the time to make real use of your talents. Learn to embrace the constraints around you and make the very best of them. Do not work longer than forty hours per week. Instead, decide to focus on your work and do it better. Satisfaction guaranteed.

Spring-clean your life

All relationships, patterns of daily living, and working practices benefit from a spring clean. Combat the staleness and boredom of mind, body and spirit by introducing fresh ideas. These could lead to physical, emotional and work stimulation and increased satisfaction.

Introduce new experiences into your personal, family and leisure life. Once your nearest and dearest get used to the idea of breaking with past habits and trying the new, you will find that relationships gradually change into more mature and beneficial forms.

Happiness can be a hobby that takes you away from day-to-day life and lifts your mood. Happy people are sociable. They contact friends just to see how they are and what they are doing. They know their own strengths and what they enjoy and are open to new experiences. These attitudes enable them to go out to others and to be creative.

SUMMARY

▶ Although there is a definite reduction in the levels of testosterone from age forty-five, in most men the effects of the andropause are more attributable to physical and psychological health than a reduction in testosterone.

▶ Addressing issues of diet, stress, personal matters and exercise has a significantly beneficial effect on the symptoms associated with the andropause.

▶ It's easy to look for a cause that can be addressed by medication, but, in most cases, it is the wrong approach and does not solve the problems.

▶ Libido and erectile dysfunction are not resolved by testosterone supplements unless the testosterone levels are very low indeed, which is seldom the case.

▶ These problems, as with many other of the symptoms, are reversible by lifestyle changes, involving diet, attention to stress issues, and exercise. As with most medical conditions, addressing the cause, rather than the effects, of a condition is a much more successful approach. So revisit the points in Chapter 1 (low-GI foods), Chapter 2 (looking after your heart), Chapter 3 (de-stressing), Chapter 4 (dealing with fat issues), Chapter 5 (taking care of your fluid intake) and Chapter 6 (being sensible about alcohol).

CHAPTER 8

How Good is Your Posture?

Correct posture forms the basis of your entire musculoskeletal system: the tone of muscles, coordination of movement and balance of muscular movement around joints. Not only that, but stable posture – in every position – can permit effective function of the internal organs by allowing their unrestricted expansion during normal physiological activities, for example blood flow, breathing and gastrointestinal function.

The musculature of the body is based on the principle that for every *agonist* muscle (or *flexor*) there is an *antagonist* (or *extensor*). This means that if you have a muscle that performs one function across a joint, you need to have a muscle performing exactly the opposite on the other side of the joint to achieve muscular stability. For example, on the upper arm the bicep muscle flexes the arm, while the tricep extends it.

Obviously the muscles on each side of the joint need to be of approximately equal power otherwise muscle imbalance occurs.

This all seems perfectly straightforward, and in theory it is. However, in practice, it is actually very difficult to achieve. The practical demonstration of muscle balance is posture. Most people think of posture as being when you are at rest, which is called *static posture*. However, posture is of essential importance at all times, whether you're at rest or in the process of movement, the latter being *dynamic posture*. So, in simple terms, we have static posture when we are at rest and dynamic posture during movement.

All muscles are dependent on the length–tension relationship of the muscle, in other words the length of the muscle compared with the amount of tension within the muscle. And obviously, as muscles operate across joints, the amount of pressure placed on the joint is dependent on the length–tension relationship. This determines not only the amount of pressure on the joint, but also (much more importantly) the alignment of the joint. If the length–tension relationship of the muscles is not carefully balanced, the constant tension between the agonist and antagonist muscles can actually age the joints prematurely, leading to joint, tendon, ligament and muscle injuries, which inevitably lead to premature arthritis. Muscle imbalance causes postural distortion.

But the most important point is that muscle balance is an intrinsic fact of body function at all times, not just at rest, and the alignment of the muscles determines the health of the joints. Once you realise and accept this principle, the damage to muscles and joints from poor posture becomes obvious.

Injuries can become cumulative through several forms of tissue trauma quite simply based on muscle imbalance. For example, muscular imbalance from poor posture can cause trauma to the tissues and inflammation, with potential intramuscular adhesions. This leads to muscle spasm and muscular imbalance, with further tissue trauma and possible further adhesions. And so you can see that a cycle of cumulative injury develops, all based on muscle imbalance, or posture, in the first instance.

And the primary cause of muscle imbalance and poor posture is a sedentary lifestyle.

Muscle imbalances actually cause trauma to the joints, which causes inflammation and, as we have seen with back pain, this can lead to muscle spasm around the joint. 'Knots' develop in the muscles. We've all experienced muscle spasm around the shoulder and neck region during periods of stress. When the muscles go into spasm, flexibility is lost and therefore the nervous system can't maintain the balance between agonist and antagonist muscles.

The more prolonged the muscular imbalance, the greater the trauma, the greater the inflammation and the greater the permanent damage.

Common muscle imbalances

Let us examine the common muscle imbalances that occur primarily as a result of a sedentary lifestyle:

- tightening of the hip flexors and the hamstring muscles

- weakening of the upper-back muscles

- hip rotation imbalance

Hip flexors and hamstring muscles

Basically, when we remain sedentary for long periods of time (such as sitting at a desk), muscles tend to contract and the antagonist muscles are overstretched for long periods of time. Look at the diagram overleaf, showing the typical position of someone seated hunched over a computer, which is a very common example of poor posture. You can clearly see that the muscles that flex the hip are contracted, those that extend the hip are stretched, and this is a frequent occurrence for many men. Muscles were meant to be at their resting length for most of the time, and not contracted or extended for long periods. When you remain seated constantly, the hip is flexed and the extensor muscles at the back are extended, sometimes for hours at a time. Quite simply, the body is designed for an upright posture, not seated, because, in the upright position

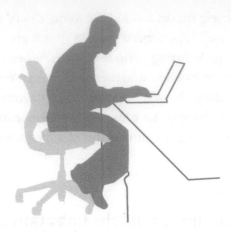

POOR POSTURE

(which may be standing but is also the normal resting position in bed), all of the muscles are at their genuine resting length, and the extensors and the flexors are of equal length and tension. Whenever we flex or extend muscles for extended periods of time, they become tight and go into spasm.

When you are seated in the same position for long periods of time, this causes maximal hip flexion of about 90 degrees, with a secondary effect on the back whereby the lower part of the spine, the lumbar spine, becomes arched and there is a resultant curvature (known as *kyphosis*) of the upper back to compensate.

Therefore, adopting an incorrect posture while sitting can cause significant back problems throughout the entire length of the back, not just the upper back and neck.

When you are sitting incorrectly for long periods of time, the main extensor muscle of the hip, the gluteus maximus, is lengthened for long periods and becomes weak. As a direct result, the hamstring muscles on the back of the upper leg become tight, weakening their action and further exacerbating the curvature of the spine.

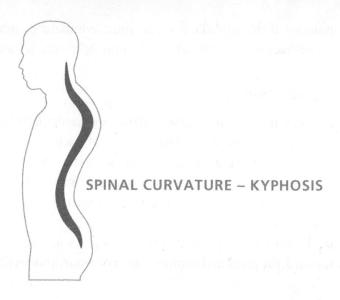

SPINAL CURVATURE – KYPHOSIS

Poor upper-back posture

Shoulder posture is absolutely crucial to the prevention of back problems, both in the upper and lower back. It is obviously tempting, when sitting for long periods when either writing or using a computer, to hunch forward, thereby placing great strain on the upper back muscles. This is of course initially precipitated by the tension in the hip flexors already described, which cause this kyphosis of the upper back in an attempt to correct the muscle imbalance.

As a result, the shoulders tend to become protracted rather than retracted, and tension develops across the upper back with the muscles going into spasm. It is obviously essential when sitting for long periods of time to ensure the correct posture, because otherwise problems in both upper and lower back are inevitable due to muscle spasm.

As an adjunct, one of the commonest mistakes that those of us who take up weight training can develop is to overexercise the muscles on the chest (pectoral muscles) by performing too many bench presses or press-ups, without placing as much emphasis on exercising the upper-back muscles, which are the antagonist muscles. If this mistake is made, muscle imbalance develops and upper-back pain, secondary to the muscle spasm, is inevitable.

Hip rotation

Let us return to the importance of posture, particularly hip position. In the prevention of the development of back pain and shoulder tightness, one of the central problems that must be addressed is the way some of us tend to sit, either with legs apart, which causes the hip to rotate externally, or with legs crossed, which causes excessive internal rotation. As the natural resting position of the body (and therefore the musculature) is upright with the toes pointing forward, the problem becomes rather obvious, as does the solution.

External hip rotation

If you sit with legs apart for excessive periods, the hip naturally tends to turn outwards, placing great strain on the muscles controlling this. But much more importantly, when the hip is in this position it is much more likely to cause pressure on the sciatic nerve, with the resultant typical sciatic pain down the back of the calf into the heel.

Internal rotation of the hip

Similarly, if the opposite seating position is maintained with the legs crossed for long periods of time, the hip is turned inwards or internally. This causes a particular imbalance in the muscles around the knee joint and can lead to increased arthritis of the knee.

How to correct postural imbalance

It's important to recognise that posture is an essential part of our health at all times, not just when we are seated at a desk. And, as with many conditions, it's better to concentrate on prevention rather than cure. The main components of prevention are the following.

- **Be aware of the problem and be prepared to address it** This may seem obvious but it is the single most important pro-active measure you can take. This is the most important point, because it is frequently ignored or becomes a mere afterthought – by which time it is usually too late.

- **Think 'muscle balance'** Muscle balance involves considering your body in its basic component form as muscles on one side of a joint with opposing muscles on the other. If you consider it this way then you will inevitably not overstretch one at the expense of the other. Always remember that the most natural position of the body is standing upright with the feet pointing forwards, and try to adopt this in most of the actions that you do. Don't place the body in abnormal positions such as sitting for long periods of the day hunched over a desk or computer. Move around, and always maintain your posture while seated.

- **Relax** Relaxation is the single most important aspect of posture. If you're not relaxed, this can be translated to the muscles as muscle tension and ultimately muscle spasm. When the muscles go into spasm, muscle balance is inevitably impaired and trauma and inflammation to the muscles and joints will follow, leading to arthritis or exacerbating a pre-existing condition.

- **Exercise carefully** It is essential to exercise in a balanced manner, never exercising one group of muscles at the expense of others, and always exercising each side of the joint equally. So, when you exercise the pectoral muscles on the front of the chest, it is essential to exercise the large latissimus dorsi and rhomboids of the upper back as well, otherwise muscle imbalance is inevitable.

- **Remember posture** Posture is with you at all times, in every position of the body, and therefore it is important to maintain acceptable body posture at all times. There is no second chance:

when posture is lost for significant periods of time, permanent damage will result that cannot be reversed.

There are many more aspects to posture than muscle balance and health. Posture can also affect aspects of your normal life. Let us look at just two major ones.

Self-esteem

Posture has an inevitable effect on your self-confidence and self-esteem. If you adopt a poor posture with hunched shoulders, which means much more looking at your toes than looking into the eyes of the person you're talking to, your self-confidence and self-esteem are significantly diminished. Much more importantly, others realise this and may take advantage accordingly.

Career

Career development, too, is directly affected by your presentation of yourself and your abilities. Irrespective of how intelligent you may be, unless you can project your abilities, they will be downgraded. So, while posture has a major effect on your own personal self-confidence and self-esteem, it also has an effect on how others perceive you. And this includes how your employer perceives your attitude. A strong posture exudes self-esteem and confidence.

SUMMARY

▶ Correct posture forms the basis of your entire musculoskeletal system: tone, power, coordination and balance.

▶ For every muscular action (agonist) there is an antagonistic muscular action.

→

▶ The key is to ensure muscular balance.

▶ Muscular imbalance causes trauma to joints.

▶ When you exercise, do so carefully.

▶ Be aware of the importance of relaxation.

▶ Posture has significant effects on mental as well as physical health. Appropriate posture can be reflected in self-esteem and confidence, while inappropriate posture may have the opposite effect, which can materially determine career development.

CHAPTER 9

Muscle Up

We men have an underlying anxiety about being and looking unfit. In the competitive, commercial world being overweight may be equated with negative personality qualities. Feeling confident in your appearance inspires confidence in others.

In general, men are obsessed with muscle tone. And this obsession reaches a pinnacle in our forties and fifties, but lack of exercise means muscle tone diminishes rapidly. Magazines are bulging with more articles about muscles than there are muscles themselves, and gym memberships abound, usually unused or underutilised. The mere act of taking out a gym membership seems to confer on some people an immediate improvement in their fitness and muscle power, despite the fact that they probably never attend!

But muscles really are very important, although not perhaps in the way that you might expect. Developing the muscular framework of the body with bodybuilding exercises is important, not just for cosmetic appearance, but also to improve capillary circulation, and, as we have discussed, for posture. To really understand this concept, we need to look at what muscle is and what it does. Unless you understand these basic principles, it is impossible to develop muscles appropriately, and equally impossible to achieve a healthy balance. While cardiovascular exercise is very useful to develop improved capillary circulation, removal of toxins by lymphatic drainage and stamina, it does not have the capability to produce the equivalent muscular balance of agonist and antagonist muscles, which can be achieved only by specific *isotonic* or *isometric* exercise – two terms we'll look at shortly.

Muscles make up about 50 per cent of your body weight – but it's not just the muscles on the outside of the body, which you can see the shape of through the skin, but also those inside, which are by far the more important. Muscles are divided into three categories:

- Skeletal. This is the type of muscle we normally think of when discussing this subject – the biceps (upper arms), the quadriceps (thighs) and abs (abdomen), for instance. More on these later.

- Smooth. Smooth muscle makes up all of the viscera, the intestines, the bladder and the muscle in internal organs.

- Cardiac. Cardiac muscle is different from all the others, as it has 'intrinsic rhythmicity'. Sounds like a blues band, but it means that cardiac muscle can actually beat on its own without nervous input. If you were to take the heart out of the body it would actually beat (provided it was supplied with oxygen and nutrition), but only at a very slow rate: 36–44 beats per minute, which is obviously insufficient for normal activity. The heart rate is controlled by the autonomic nervous system for all normal functions above that level.

All of these muscles need to be taken care of for health reasons, and particularly when we reach the age of forty, as that is the age that deterioration starts to occur.

We will examine the skeletal muscle last, as that seems the most obvious muscle to exercise for health, and will first look at smooth muscle and cardiac muscle, which are equally important.

Smooth muscle

Smooth muscle makes up most of the involuntary muscles in the body such as the oesophagus (the food tube leading into the stomach), the stomach, the intestines and many other anatomical functions. How on earth can you exercise such musculature when you cannot even control it? Actually, quite simply. The first and most important principle is that all of the musculature in the body needs the same things as every other cell: food and oxygen. These come in the form of nutrition from your diet and good profusion, or blood flow, to the tissues, which is improved by preventing constriction of arteries by cholesterol and nervous function (stress), discussed in Chapter 3.

The second important point is that smooth muscle needs stimulation and this comes from roughage. We don't actually think about moving the food along our intestine. The intestine does this automatically, and it is stimulated to do this by something stretching the muscles. In other words, if you have roughage in your diet (like that provided by indigestible materials such as green plants), this stretches the muscle fibres and helps to press the food through the bowel. If you don't have roughage in your diet, the bowel isn't stimulated and it becomes dormant.

And this is the major cause of bowel cancer. The single most important feature in preventing bowel cancer, which can come on in our fifties in men, is a diet with lots of roughage. If the diet also includes good nutrition and high levels of antioxidants, this is a further preventive measure against bowel cancer. Simply have a salad with your steak and you are going to cut your risk of bowel cancer dramatically.

The second major factor in exercising smooth muscle in the bowel and preventing bowel cancer is water, because bowel motions need lubrication. We simply don't drink enough of it. This was explained in detail in Chapter 5, where we discussed the importance of fluid balance. But the basic principle is to drink on a regular basis – not just when you feel thirsty but also at times when you don't think you need to drink. This keeps the contractor muscle of the bowel moving, prevents constipation and prevents many of the typical diseases that occur in middle age such as cancer (obviously), irritable bowel syndrome, colitis and peptic ulcers.

Cardiac muscle

Although the heart is a very specialised form of muscle, performing an essential function for life, it is still a muscle and has all the needs and requirements of other muscles:

- nutrition (from the arteries)
- oxygen (from the arteries)
- the removal of toxic waste products (via the veins)

Cardiac muscle, then, has the same need for a blood flow to provide its nutrition and oxygen and to remove its waste products as everywhere else in the body, and therefore is subject to the same problems when that blood flow is blocked. This is explained in considerable detail in Chapter 2, but it is worth emphasising at this point that the essential difference between cardiac muscle and any other form of muscle is that, if we don't maintain that blood flow constantly for any period of time, the cardiac muscle will die (through myocardial infarction or heart attack) – and so will we. So this is probably the single most important muscle in the body to maintain, and the way to do it is explained clearly in Chapter 2.

Skeletal muscle

Skeletal muscle is the substance that we all *think* of as muscle, as it sits on the surface of the skeleton. This is not particularly surprising, as there are an awful lot of muscles there: about 260 pairs of muscles and 5 single muscles. It is important to understand how the musculature works, otherwise exercises can be distinctly dangerous rather than helpful.

The reason why we mostly have pairs of muscles rather than single muscles is that, for every muscle action, there has to be an opposite muscle reaction. In other words, for every agonist muscle there has to be an antagonist action. We saw this earlier but it's worth repeating, because if this principle is not strictly followed muscular imbalance occurs, which has significant consequences for posture and health. So, if you exercise one particular muscle, you must exercise the opposite muscle to the same degree.

The why and how of exercising

The most obvious thing that drives most of us to exercise is because we want to look better and feel better – and we often emphasise the former. But the most important reason to exercise is that it improves the *profusion* (the blood flow) to the muscles, taking oxygen and nutrition to them and removing the toxic waste products, which are a major component in disease and ageing. In addition, exercise improves the blood flow *throughout the whole of the body* – tissues as well as muscles.

Now you understand *why* we are exercising, let's discuss *how* to exercise. That would seem rather obvious, as we simply move muscles and they become larger, but it is not as simple as that, and you really need to understand the process before commencing, otherwise you can do yourself serious harm.

Many popular men's magazines are full of exercises demonstrating healthy young men with abdominal six-packs and biceps the size of tree trunks. This is all very well, but it is neither reasonable nor natural. And it is certainly not feasible for men in their forties and fifties, unless you have a tremendous amount of time to spend (waste?) trying to achieve the impossible.

Before describing what you need to do to be healthy in a 'muscle-up' programme, it is first essential to describe what you must *not* do.

Don't take up jogging

Jogging is an excellent form of exercise when you are fit, and an excellent way of precipitating a heart attack when you're not. If you are overweight and under-muscled (as most of us are in our forties) jogging is just a complicated way of destroying your hip and knee joints and placing a tremendous strain on your heart and lungs. This is not to say that you cannot take up jogging later when you have lost weight and have muscled up, but not at the beginning.

Although there are many advantages to joining a gym, provided it has appropriate programmes available, there is no advantage in immediately starting to spend hours on the treadmill – or pumping iron. This is another typical male attitude to the overweight/under-muscled physique, and it normally comes on about 1 January of every year. Joining a gym can be expensive and unnecessary. The secret is to become reasonably fit first, and then make the decision as to whether you wish to expand your exercise programme to more extreme lengths.

Don't go on a crash diet

As you will have realised, this programme enables your intake of high-quality protein to be almost unlimited, which means that you will be replenishing the protein that your body needs to build muscle. If you go on a crash, low-calorie diet within twenty-four hours the body will start to break down body protein (in preference to fat) and all that will happen is that you will become weaker and more susceptible to illness and infection.

Now that we have described what not to do, we can proceed with what you need to do. It's important to start slowly. With that basic principle understood, you can start to exercise healthily and safely. A safe exercise programme consists of two parts:

■ isometric exercises

■ isotonic exercises

Exercise mythology – the facts

Before we describe the exercises, let us dispel a few dangerous myths about exercise.

Myth 1: You need to exercise for at least an hour per day, three times a week for it to be effective

This is simply not true. The *most effective* form of exercise is undoubtedly walking for twenty minutes three times a week. Surprising though this may seem, it has the most significant effect on improving capillary circulation to the tissues in terms of effort expended. Of course, that doesn't mean that more exercise isn't likely to be more effective – it certainly will be – but 'too much too soon' is dangerous. We will be describing exercises that you can actually perform while sitting that are very effective, and can be done every day in just a few moments.

Myth 2: Exercise burns fat

Exercise in isolation, without addressing the nutritional aspects, does not burn fat. Of course, when you exercise you require an energy source, but as we exercise we increase our insulin levels and insulin actually prevents us from burning fat. If you do exercise extremely hard, you will need to have tremendous will power to prevent the ravenous hunger that follows thereafter, so that is simply not an option. A much simpler solution is to reduce the insulin in your diet by dietary changes, and then, with lowered insulin, exercise will burn fat. But, for the most effective solution to burning fat, combine an insulin-

→

lowering, non-calorie-counting diet with an effective muscle-training regime.

Myth 3: No pain, no gain

This is a simple recipe for developing a heart attack. We cannot think of worse advice to give someone who is overweight than to suggest that they exercise to the point of developing pain.

And this leads us on to the obvious question of 'What *is* pain during exercise?' Basically exercise falls into two separate phases: aerobic and anaerobic. In the first form we are using oxygen for our tissues and the muscles to develop; in the second form there isn't enough oxygen and the muscles develop a substance called *lactic acid*, which causes pain. So you can see that pain is actually the body's way of telling you that you have done enough and to stop. 'No pain, no gain' is just a simple way of putting excess stress on your heart and causing problems.

So you can now understand why you should never exercise to the point of experiencing pain, as this is telling you that there is not enough oxygen in your muscles to continue.

How to exercise effectively: isotonic versus isometric

Having described what you must not do, we now go back to the isometric and isotonic exercises. To follow this programme you need to perform a series of exercises that are isometric, but you don't necessarily need to proceed to Phase Two, which are the isotonic exercises.

While isotonic exercises are those in which the muscles move (as in weight training), *isometric* exercises are those in which the muscles don't move. We can appreciate you are now considering that this is becoming rather complicated. First, we have explained that you can eat as many calories as you like, provided they are not refined carbohydrates, and you will lose fat and weight, and now we are telling you that you can exercise your muscles without moving.

But this is not a form of madness: it's actually a well-established exercise programme performed by most Olympic athletes. Let me explain exactly what we mean.

When you contract a muscle (using your biceps, for instance, to lift a dumbbell) the muscle shortens and, by holding that position over a period of time, this will cause the muscle fibres to increase and the muscle will increase tone.

This would seem the most effective way of exercising. But the body doesn't work in that way, and muscles develop their maximal power at resting length, rather than moving. This means that if you contract both the agonist and antagonist muscles at the same time, the net result will be no movement, but the muscles will still be contracting massively.

This may seem difficult to understand when expressed in writing, but it is very simple in practice. For example, let us demonstrate how this can exercise the pectoral muscles (pectoralis major and pectoralis minor) in a way that will be very simple to explain, and you will feel the benefit almost immediately. Place both hands in front of you, with your elbows bent and palms together about 15–20 cm from your chest (see diagram opposite).

Take in a breath of about half your lungs' capacity (in other words, not a full breath) and, while holding your breath, press both hands together as firmly as you are able for about ten seconds, then relax. What you have done is to compress the pectoralis major and pectoralis minor (the main muscles of the chest) and cause the fibres to start to increase in size. You will actually feel the difference as you do this, and you will feel the difference in increasing amounts every day. What will happen is that the tone of the muscles will increase on a daily basis and, as the fat over the muscles decreases, their appearance will be much more in keeping with what you want.

But of course, as we saw earlier in this chapter, all agonist muscles have an antagonist, which you must exercise at the same time. So, if we exercise the pectoral muscles, we need then to exercise the back muscles that act against this movement to balance the musculature of the body. Once again, this is simply performed. Stand with your back to a chair (such as a dining chair), placing both hands behind your back and grasping the sides of the chair.

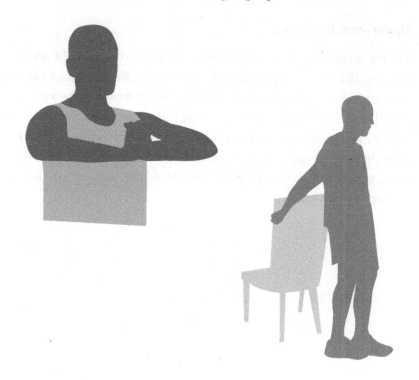

Take in a half-breath and hold. Press both hands inwards, as if trying to compress the chair as firmly as possible. Do this without relaxation for ten seconds and relax. Once again, you will feel the immediate effect of the contraction of the back muscles, and within a month you will actually feel much more toned and healthy.

Daily ten-minute isometric exercise routine

We'll now look at a series of isometric exercises covering most of the major muscles groups of the body and taking no more than 8–10 minutes a day.

Upper-arm exercises

Having reduced the subcutaneous (beneath the skin) fat layer that covers the muscles, we need to improve the tone of the muscles to provide the desired muscular contour to the biceps and triceps.

Upper-arm Exercise 1

For the biceps, bend your left arm in front of you to a right angle, keeping the elbow approximately level with the waist and place your right hand over your left wrist and grasp firmly. Take a moderate breath, and hold, and at the same time press up with your left arm while pressing down with your right. In this position, the left arm should not move during the period of flexion against resistance, with a net no-movement result. Hold the tension for about ten seconds and relax.

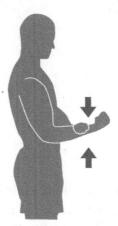

Repeat this on the right side to exercise the right bicep, once again ensuring that the arms do not move.

Upper-arm Exercise 2

Having exercised the agonist, or flexor, muscle (the biceps), we then need to exercise the antagonist, or extensor, muscle (the triceps). This time we are going to use the same motion, bending your arm to a right angle, but this time placing your right hand *under* your left wrist to grasp. Take in a moderate breath and hold, and press down with your left arm while resisting movement with your right, hold for about ten seconds and then relax.

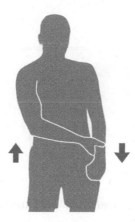

Repeat this movement on the right side to exercise the right triceps muscle in the same manner.

Shoulder exercises

Most men don't realise that it is actually the shoulders that give the upper body its characteristic shape. There is always a concentration on waist and chest exercises, but the rotator cup of the shoulder holds the upper limb girdle in place, so it is important to exercise these muscles.

The shoulder joint has a wider range of movement than any other. There are many muscles around the rotator cuff of the shoulder. However, the deltoid muscle surrounds the shoulder cuff and it is important to exercise all movements of the deltoid to avoid muscle imbalance.

The beauty of these exercises is that they exercise all muscle groups at the same time. If you improve the tone of the shoulder muscles, posture improves, body profile improves and health improves. And you require no more than an open doorway to perform the entire exercise routine.

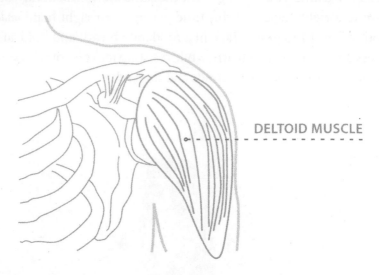

DELTOID MUSCLE

Shoulder Exercise 1: deltoids and supraspinatus

Stand in an open doorway and place both hands against the upper lintel. Take in a moderate breath, hold it, and press upwards as hard as you can for about ten seconds, before relaxing. This exercises the muscles that raise the shoulders and hold the rotator cuff in place.

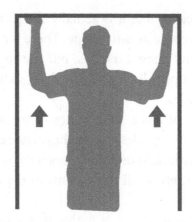

Shoulder Exercise 2: deltoids and teres major

Standing in the open doorway, make a fist with both hands and place the outer edges of your hands against the sides of the doorway. Once again, take in a moderate breath and hold it, pressing as hard as you can against the door supports for about ten seconds before relaxing. This exercises the muscles on the outer part of the shoulder, which gives the shoulders their characteristic roundness.

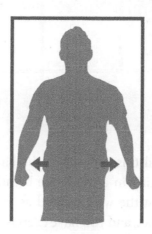

To balance all of these actions, you need to exercise the muscles on the front and the back of the shoulder, and to do this you need a wall and nothing else.

Shoulder Exercise 3: deltoids, front

Stand facing a wall, about 10 cm away, make a fist with both hands and place the leading edges of the fists against the wall, taking in a moderate breath and holding it (see page 134). Press as hard as you can against the wall for about ten seconds and relax. This exercises the muscles on the front of the shoulder.

Shoulder Exercise 4: deltoids, rear

To exercise the muscles (the antagonist muscles) on the rear part of the shoulder, stand with your back against the wall. Make a fist

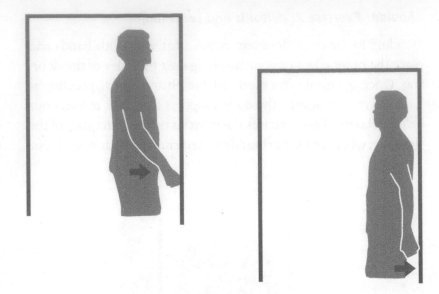

with both hands and this time place the back edges of the fists against the wall, taking in a moderate breath and holding, then pressing back against the wall as hard as you can for about ten seconds as usual. Relax, and you have exercised the muscles on the rear of the shoulders.

It is important to exercise all of these muscle groups, and not just any individual muscle. These muscles are balanced in a very delicate manner, and not just the ones you can see but the ones under the surface; and, if you don't complete all of the exercise routine, it can be very dangerous, causing muscle imbalance.

Exercising the back muscles

Surprising as it may seem, you can actually exercise the back muscles, too, without moving from your own room or using any specialist equipment.

Exercise of the back muscles (which are the support of the body) is essential for posture and for muscular balance throughout the body. Never exercise the chest muscles without concurrently exercising those of the back – a common mistake – otherwise serious muscular imbalance will develop: the back muscles are the antagonists of the chest and abdominal muscles. However, it is essential to emphasise that if you have back problems you should be very careful about performing back exercises at any time and should take advice from your physician before proceeding.

Back Exercise 1: upper back

The first muscle is the 'lats', or latissimus dorsi. This is the powerful back muscle that gives the V shape that is so desirable. The exercise is performed sitting down and hardly moving.

Sit on a dining chair (or desk chair) facing a table or desk. Place both hands palms down on the table or desk, taking in a moderate breath as usual, and press down firmly on the surface for about ten seconds while holding your breath.

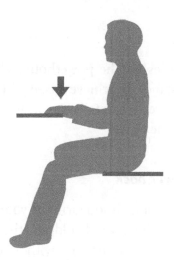

Back Exercise 2: upper back

Take a small towel, stand upright with feet about shoulder width apart, and hold the towel about shoulder width above your head. Take a moderate breath and hold. Grasp the towel tightly with both hands and try to pull both arms outwards and downwards away from one another. Hold for about ten seconds and relax.

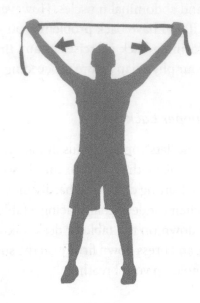

The lower back

The lower-back muscles are the powerhouse of the body. They control posture and stance. To achieve this requires a very complex series of muscles in three separate layers arranged in an intricate pattern behind the spine.

Back Exercise 3: lower back

Lie face down on the floor with your arms by your sides (see opposite). Take in a moderate breath and hold, and then raise your head and shoulders about 10 cm off the floor without using your arms. Hold this position for about ten seconds and then relax.

Back Exercise 4: lower back

To exercise the remaining lower-back muscles, once again lie face down on the floor but this time with legs and arms extended outwards. Take in a moderate breath, hold and arch your back backwards while trying to lift both arms and legs off the ground. Hold for ten seconds then relax.

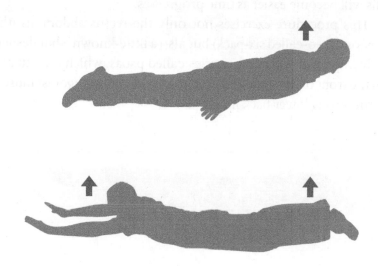

The abdomen

Having exercised the lower-back muscles, we turn to the antagonist muscles, the abdominal muscles. In most people, the abdominal muscles have endured years of inertia, so they are usually some of the weakest on the body. So start slowly and gradually increase as the muscle tone improves. Any overexertion of the abdominal muscles at this stage will cause significant damage, and even possible hernias.

Abdominal Exercise

Lie flat on your back with your hands by your sides. Raise both legs off the ground keeping the legs straight, and hold for about ten seconds. You should raise them only about 5–6 cm to obtain the maximum tension. Relax after about ten seconds and slowly lower the legs to the ground. If you can't hold for ten seconds, hold for a few seconds and release, but do not hold to the extent of having pain. The abdominal muscles will gradually increase in tone and this will become easier as time progresses.

This procedure exercises not only the rectus abdominis (the 'abs' or the so-called six-pack) but also a little-known – but desperately important – pair of muscles called psoas, which are situated on the front of the spine and act as a very potent antagonist muscle to the strong lower-back musculature.

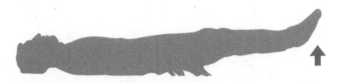

The legs

Once again, for these exercises all we require is a door frame and a wall.

Leg Exercise 1

To exercise the muscles on the front of the leg (quadriceps), stand in an open door frame with your back against one doorpost, lift one leg and place it against the other doorpost.

Take a moderate breath and hold. Brace your back against the doorpost, and press against the other doorpost with your foot as hard as you can for about ten seconds, then relax. Repeat the exercise with the other leg.

This not only improves the tone of quadriceps on the front of the leg, but also the calf muscles, which are trying to extend the foot. Obviously, having exercised the quadriceps, we need to exercise the hamstrings on the back of the leg (and also the buttocks).

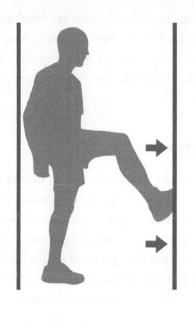

Leg Exercise 2

Standing with your back to a wall, with both shoulders and heels resting against the wall, place the palms of both hands flat against the wall. Take in a moderate breath and press your right heel as hard as you can against the wall for about ten seconds and relax. The tightening of the muscles will be felt immediately. Repeat the exercise with the left leg.

The neck

Having completed most of the obvious muscles of the body, we now need to do neck exercises. This is an area commonly forgotten. However, it's one of the most important areas, because the neck is a major form of weakness with usually poor musculature holding up the head, and the vertebrae that hold the head can develop problems in the intervertical spaces, causing pain, which can translate down to the arms in later life (cervical spondulosis). So exercises for the neck will undoubtedly improve your chances of not developing arthritis later in life. It will also improve the cosmetic appearance of the neck, which can be a problem in our forties.

Neck Exercise 1: forward/backward

Place your palms on the front of the forehead, take a moderate breath and hold. While pressing forward with your forehead, press backwards with your hands to maintain a steady position with no movement. Hold for approximately ten seconds and then relax. To counteract this we need to exercise the antagonist muscles on the back of the neck and to do so we simply place the palms of both hands on the back of the head, and after taking a moderate breath and holding, push the head backwards against the palms while pushing forward with the palms. Release after about ten seconds.

Neck Exercise 2: lateral

Place your right palm against the right side of the head, take in a moderate breath and hold, pressing with your head against your palm and palm against the head, holding the head motionless for about ten seconds before relaxing. Repeat the exercise on the left side.

Neck Exercise 3: rotational

Rotate your head in a circular motion from left to right. Repeat the movement nine times then perform the same exercise with a circular movement from right to left.

This completes the isometric exercise programme, and you should be able to perform this in less than 10 minutes on a daily basis with no equipment, either in your office or in the privacy of your own

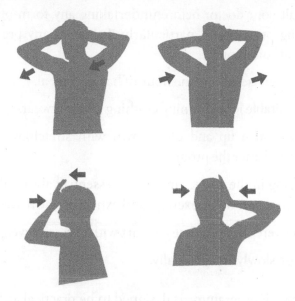

home. It is absolutely essential to complete an exercise programme which is isometric, coupled with a walking programme, for health. This is safe and will cause no injuries but will improve the tone of the muscles, enhancing the cosmetic appearance, and also significantly improving blood flow to the muscles and the removal of toxic wastes.

The next stage is an isotonic programme, which is entirely discretionary. If you perform this programme you will undoubtedly look better and feel better, but it is not essential.

Isotonic exercises

In this section, we are going to deal with basic weight training in a practical and sensible way. As explained earlier, it is not necessary to perform weight training, but it is essential to perform the isometric exercises. Before commencing any form of weight training, however, you must adhere to several basic rules, which never vary.

- Consult your doctor before undertaking any form of weight-training programme, particularly if there is any pre-existing medical condition.

- Never exercise within one hour of having a meal.

- Wear suitable loose training clothing and footwear.

- Always warm up and cool down with stretching exercises before and after the programme.

- Breathing in the correct manner is essential: always inhale on the easiest part of the exercise and exhale on the hardest part.

- Never overexercise and never start with excessive weight.

- Exercise slowly and gradually.

The following programme is designed to be practical and simple. If you wish to follow an extensive weight-training programme where you spend hours per week, then this is not for you. On the contrary, it is meant to be a very efficient programme that will take no more than ten minutes per day, four days per week. Equally, it exercises all of the main muscle groups but obviously you can't exercise absolutely everything in ten minutes. It is intended to give you a sleek, toned body, not some large muscle-bound appearance – in other words, to exaggerate the normal contours of the body, but not excessively.

Stretching exercises

In this section, as in the later sections, it is important to exercise and to stretch all of the main muscle groups before beginning.

Stretching Exercise 1: chest

Clasp your hands together behind your back (see opposite, top). Keeping the arms straight, lift the arms as high as possible to stretch, and hold for ten seconds, then relax.

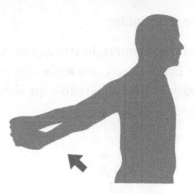

Stretching Exercise 2: upper back

Stretch your right hand across behind your back and grip the right wrist with the left hand (see below, left). Pull down with your right wrist and hold for ten seconds, then relax. Repeat on the other side.

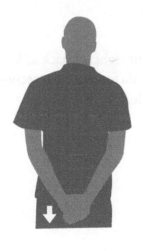

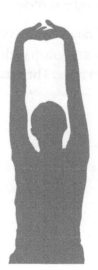

Stretching Exercise 3: lower back

Raise both hands above your head and clasp them together. Try to reach as high as you can, holding the contraction for ten seconds, then relax.

Stretching Exercise 4: shoulder

Stretch your right hand and your right arm across your chest at the level of the shoulder. Flex your left arm across the right upper arm or elbow and pull back as hard as possible for about ten seconds and then relax. Repeat for the left arm.

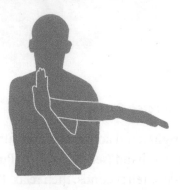

Stretching Exercise 5: quadriceps

Stand straight with feet together. Flex your right leg back as far as possible and grasp with the right hand. Hold for about ten seconds and then relax. Then repeat on the left side.

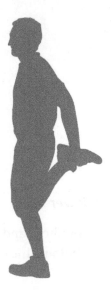

Stretching Exercise 6: hamstring

Extend your right leg out as far as possible, straight with the heel to the ground. Bend forward at the waist, feeling the tension on the leg and hold for about ten seconds, then relax. Repeat with the left leg.

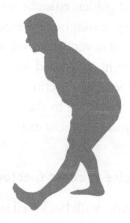

Having now performed these basic but essential stretching exercises, to prevent any possible muscle injury, we can proceed with the short programme. This will be divided into the major muscle groups:

- chest
- upper back
- lower back
- abdominal muscles
- arm
- leg

In these exercises, we are going to use a weights machine such as a multi-gym. We appreciate that these are available only in some homes or in gyms, but the reason we advise a machine is that they are much safer than using dumbbells or barbells for the first time.

Just to reiterate, there is no need to perform isotonic exercise to achieve muscle tone. However, if you wish to, this is the safest way of doing it. The simplest form of isotonic exercise, which we certainly advocate, is either walking for thirty minutes three times per week, or swimming for thirty minutes twice a week.

Your weight-training programme

Remember to follow the golden rules of warming up, wear loose clothing and avoid excessive weights. If weight training is a new experience, start low. You can never be too low with weights, so always begin on the lowest weight suggested for each exercise. Perform the exercises with the specified repetitions for a minimum of two weeks before increasing the weight by the next increment. Of course, if you are experienced, you will know exactly how to proceed.

Weight-training Exercise 1: chest (pectorals)

Sit on the weights machine, with back well supported, add approximately 30–45 kg initially and press forward against the resistance slowly. Return the weight back to the rest position slowly. Perform ten times, then rest.

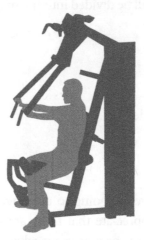

Once again, sitting comfortably on the weights machine with back well supported, place the elbows at right angles on the support and press forward, bringing the elbows together before gradually releasing the tension slowly. Do not let go. To release the tension slowly is as much of an exercise for the chest muscles as the initial thrust. Once again, perform ten times at approximately 30–45 kg and relax.

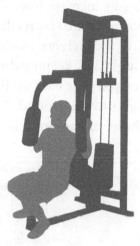

Weight-training Exercise 2: upper back (latissimus dorsi)

Seated on the weights machine, set approximately 50–60 kg of weights and extend both arms upwards to grasp the bar. Pull the bar down behind the neck and slowly allow the bar to regain the upper position. Once again, perform ten times and relax.

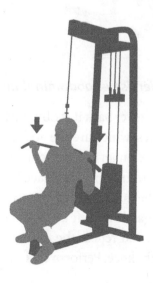

Weight-training Exercise 3: lower back

Once again, do not use excessive weights initially. This is an exercise that can undoubtedly increase lower-back muscle, but can equally damage it if not performed correctly.

Standing in front of the weights machine, grasp the bar at approximately knee height and, keeping the feet together and the back straight, slowly extend your back until you are upright, then slowly lower the weights to the ground. Perform ten times and relax. This exercises the lower-back muscles tremendously.

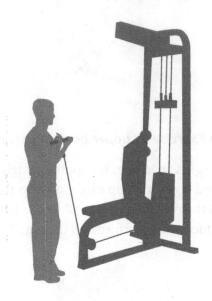

Weight-training Exercise 4: abdominal muscles

Having exercised the lower back it is obviously essential to exercise the antagonist muscles, which are the abdominal muscles.

For this exercise, lie on an incline bench with both legs straight and ankles under the restraining bar. Place both hands behind your head, and interlock the fingers. Slowly bend from the waist, touching the right elbow against the left knee. Then gradually relax until lying flat once again, and repeat the exercise by touching the left elbow against the right knee. Perform this exercise up to 5–7 times, if possible, but do not cause pain. Once again, if you're not accustomed to these exercises, they can certainly cause damage rather than improvement initially, and the secret is to progress slowly.

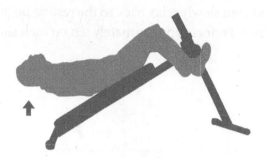

The shoulders

It is essential to exercise all of the rotator cuff muscles around the shoulder girdle. Exercises for the upper arm and the shoulder muscles are the only ones in which we use dumbbells, because they are safe in this position.

Weight-training Exercise 5: outer shoulder cuff

Place approximately 5 kg of weights on each dumbbell, and stand upright, holding the dumbbells at the side. Keeping the arm straight, raise the right arm outwards as far as possible and then slowly relax; then repeat on the left side. Do this approximately ten times.

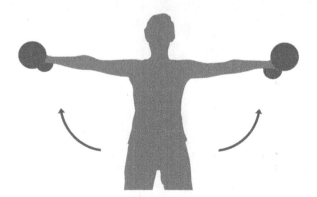

Weight-training Exercise 6: front of shoulder

Once again, holding the dumbbells by your sides, standing upright, slowly, with the arm straight, extend the right arm forward as far as possible and then slowly relax back to the resting position. Repeat on the left side. Perform approximately ten on each side.

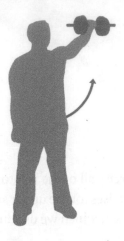

Weight-training Exercise 7: rear of shoulder

Once again, standing upright with your arms by your sides, slowly extend the right arm backwards as far as possible, hold for one second, then slowly bring the arm back to the side. Perform ten times and repeat on the left side.

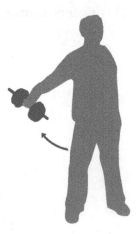

Weight-training Exercise 8: upper arm (biceps – flexors)

These exercises are known to everyone, and should be performed with not too much weight. Once again, placing approximately 10 kg on each bar, hold the dumbbells by your sides standing upright. Slowly flex both arms, keeping the elbows by your side until they reach an angle of approximately 60 degrees, then slowly relax the contraction. Perform a further nine repetitions.

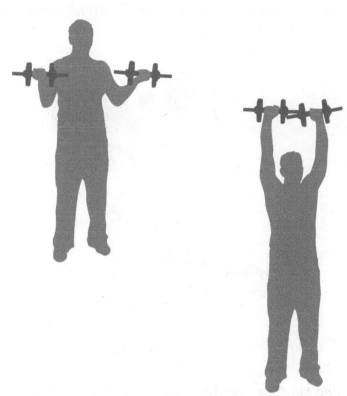

Weight-training Exercise 9: upper arm (triceps – extensors)

Once again, with approximately 10 kg on each dumbbell, hold the weights at approximately shoulder height, with elbows either side. Slowly extend both arms as high as possible then relax back to the resting position at shoulder height. Perform a further nine repetitions.

Weight-training Exercise 10: lower limb muscles (quadriceps – extensors)

Sitting on the weight machine with the back well supported, place both ankles behind the lower leg extensor bar. The weight should be no more than 45 kg initially but this can be increased as the power increases. Slowly extend both legs, then, equally slowly, return them to the resting position. You should feel the tension on the quadriceps muscles on the front of the thighs immediately. Do this ten times and relax.

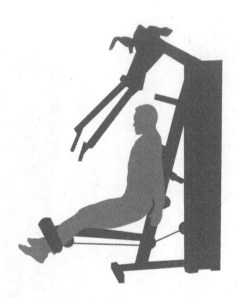

Stepping Machine Exercise: lower limb muscles (calf muscles and hamstrings – extensors)

This is performed on the stepping machine with initially very little resistance, gradually increasing as weeks progress. Stand on the stepping machine, supporting the arms by grasping the bar (see opposite). Commence stepping, alternating the right and the left legs, feeling the tension on the rear of the calves and hamstrings. Do a hundred, then relax.

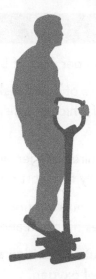

For the first four weeks, this programme of exercise should be performed for no more than two consecutive days, relax for a day, then a further two days. In other words, you are performing approximately four to five days of exercise per week only. The rest periods are essential to allow the body to recover and not over-train, particularly in the early stages when you are almost certainly using muscles that haven't been exercised for many years.

And bear in mind that, although these exercises are designed to train specific muscle groups, many other muscles are being exercised at the same time. For example, as you exercise your lower-back muscles, it is a necessary requirement to flex the abdominal muscles, which act as antagonists, in that particular position. So each of these exercises affects not just a specific group but involves all of the other fixating muscles at the same time.

The golden rule is: do not overtrain. The 'no pain, no gain' maxim is for those wishing for a heart attack.

SUMMARY

▶ Muscle comprises 50 per cent of body weight.

▶ There are three types of muscle: skeletal, smooth and cardiac, each of which has distinct and unique characteristics.

▶ Skeletal muscle requires oxygen and energy, but can function anaerobically for short periods.

▶ Smooth muscle, the musculature of the internal organs and the gut, requires nutrition and water.

▶ Cardiac muscle requires nutrition and is very susceptible to lack of oxygen.

▶ Ignore the clichés: 'exercise burns fat'; 'no pain, no gain'.

▶ An effective exercise programme involves both isotonic (where muscles actually move) and isometric (where muscles are static during maximal contraction) components.

▶ Muscles can be trained at home without the need for equipment, but, for the isotonic exercises, a weights machine is advisable.

10

Improve Your Food Awareness

Before we can discuss an 'awareness' of food, we obviously need to answer the basic question: what is food?

This might seem a relatively simple question to answer, but is it? Consider the matter for a moment: can you provide a clear definition of exactly what food is? Food is obviously something that we can purchase or grow, and that we can eat to provide us with some form of nutrition. The dictionary defines food as 'something that animals eat, or plants absorb, to keep them alive'.

Perhaps the more important question is not 'What is food?' but rather 'What is *real* food?' And by far the best definition we have ever heard for 'real food' is that given by our colleague Dr David Reilly, consultant physician, in his highly motivating, internationally acclaimed WEL programme. He describes food as 'something which you can eat for nutrition which is alive or was alive until recently'. We would add something to reflect the fact that food is best when it has not been tampered with. So our definition of real food is 'something that can be consumed for nutrition, which is alive or was alive until recently and which has not been artificially modified by man'.

Consider this for a moment, because nutrition (from food) is essential for health, and it is accorded less importance than virtually everything else in our daily lives. This definition of real food is basically that all forms of fresh meat, poultry, fish and shellfish are 'real' food, as are all forms of fresh vegetables and fruits. Eggs, cheese and dairy produce also fall into this category.

But perhaps it's best for a moment to consider those foods that are excluded from the definition of 'real food'. Foods such as cereals, flour and other grain products would, by definition, be excluded. Bread, pasta, rice and all forms of dried carbohydrate foods automatically fall outside the definition. Bread, pasta and rice, in the forms presented to you, have never been alive. They are examples of how man has artificially modified the food: the flour in bread has been ground so finely that it has a very high GI; pasta is 73 per cent dried, refined carbohydrates; and, apart from wholegrain rice, most rice consumed has the husk removed, which is the only component of the grain containing nutrients. In fact, most of those foods considered the 'basic staples' of your daily diet are excluded from the definition of 'real' food. This definition also excludes all forms of processed foods, particularly those with additives, colorants, taste enhancers and preservatives. So the old adage 'fresh food is healthiest' is true.

Let us examine this in detail, to check whether it is factually accurate. Food consists of five main categories: carbohydrates, fats, protein, vitamins and minerals. Of course the additional component to food and by far the most important is water.

Carbohydrates

The word 'carbohydrate' means sugar. All carbohydrates simply consist of sugar molecules joined together. That's right. When you eat a 'carbohydrate' what you are consuming is sugar. Now you wouldn't consider eating a bowl of sugar for breakfast but that is virtually what you *are* eating when you have a bowl of cereal or slices of toast. A typical bowl of cereal is about 75 per cent carbohydrate – without added sugar – and this equates to 75 per cent sugar, or, in more graphic terms, the equivalent of 8 teaspoons.

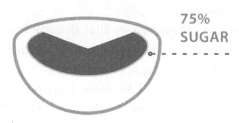

75%
SUGAR

And the next important fact to realise is that you don't need carbohydrates for health. In other words, carbohydrates are not essential for health and are not essential in your diet. Of course, although carbohydrates are not essential for health, there are obvious differences between the refined carbs in bread, pasta and rice – which have effectively no nutrients – and the unrefined carbs in fruit and vegetables, which have many other nutrients in the form of vitamins and minerals. This may seem very strange given the plethora of medical advice that carbohydrate should form a major part of a healthy 'balanced' diet. However, the medical fact is that carbohydrates are not essential for life in any way, shape or form. Carbohydrates can only provide energy, and this can be provided by alternative – and healthier – sources, such as proteins or fats, without the need for carbohydrates. We are often asked, 'How can you possibly obtain energy without carbohydrates?' To which our simple (if not rather blasé) reply is, 'That spotted cat that runs at 80 miles an hour – called the cheetah – has never eaten a sandwich, or a carbohydrate, in its life.' We appreciate that is rather simplistic, and we are certainly not cheetahs. However, the principle remains the same: unlike proteins and fats, there is no carbohydrate 'essential' to our existence, and that is certainly an indisputable medical fact.

As we saw in Chapter 1, carbohydrates breaking down into sugars stimulate the production of the hormone insulin, which in turn not only stimulates the development of fat and prevents its breakdown: it also increases cholesterol and triglyceride levels in the bloodstream, which inevitably leads to heart disease. In other words, excess carbohydrates in your diet lead to increased risk of coronary disease.

That is certainly not to say that all carbohydrates are bad: those present naturally in their unrefined state in fresh vegetables are a healthy form of energy. However, the refined carbohydrates – those heavily 'influenced' by man, such as those present in bread, pasta and rice – have a very high glycaemic index and a very high likelihood of causing raised insulin levels and an increased risk of diabetes and heart disease.

Fats

Fats have certainly had a very bad press over many years, particularly in regard to heart disease, most of which is completely inaccurate and untrue. Fats make up an essential part of our diet, but it is important to realise which fats are healthy and which are not. Fats are made up of building blocks called *fatty acids*. Certain fatty acids are essential for life, and the ones that we really need to have are omega-3 fatty acids and omega-6 fatty acids.

Omega-3 fatty acids

These are present in particularly high concentration in oily fish, such as salmon, mackerel, herring, sardines and tuna, and obviously in the fish oils that are derived from them. They are present in much lesser amounts in egg yolks, nuts and flaxseed oil.

Omega-6 fatty acids

Not as common in animal products (except egg yolks), these are found especially in seeds and their oils (particularly safflower, sesame and sunflower), vegetable oils and wholegrains. To a lesser degree, they are also present in borage, which is a very useful (and much ignored) herb in cooking.

The importance of balance in essential fats

The importance of essential fatty acids is not only that they are required to be present in the diet, but *they are required in the correct proportions to one another*. And this exemplifies the problem with the food consumed due to our lifestyles – and the almost insignificant emphasis placed on food. The correct proportion of fatty acids in your diet is approximately 2:1 for omega-6 to omega-3. Unfortunately, modern lifestyles place an emphasis on 'fast' and quickly available food, usually processed, and most processed foods contain a large amount of vegetable oils (such as corn oil), which are very high in omega-6. In many cases this can increase the proportion of omega-6 to omega-3 to 30:1, rather than the ideal of 2:1. This is certainly not healthy, and can lead to significant nutritional problems. So you can see that the definition of food as 'something that is alive or was alive until recently' is entirely correct. Although cornflower oil is perfectly healthy in isolation, when it is incorporated in large quantities into processed foods such as margarine, cakes, pastries and even meat products, the ratio of the essential fatty acids becomes grossly imbalanced, which is the antithesis of health.

Trans fats – the real killers

However, the fats that are really dangerous are trans fats. These are fats that have been created entirely by a manmade process and do not exist anywhere in nature. Fats in nature are solid but they need to be more liquid for the food industry. To achieve this unnatural state, a stream of hydrogen ions is directed at a fat to make it softer (as in many margarines and processed foods such as cakes and pastries). These trans fats are very dangerous, because they can infiltrate the walls of the normal cells of the body, thereby weakening the natural strength of the cell structure, which promotes the potential development of various diseases – and certainly advances the ageing process. Once again, fresh food (without the intervention of man) is best and those foods that man creates are inevitably unhealthy.

Proteins

The word *protein* comes from the Greek word *proteus*, which means 'first', and this is the first of all foods. Proteins are basically the building blocks of life. Most of the structure of the human body consists of pure protein. What happens is that every protein in nature, whether it is from an animal or vegetable source, breaks down into a series of component parts called *amino acids*. When we consume proteins, the body breaks them down, then absorbs the amino acids through the wall of the bowel and re-forms them as the proteins of the body: skin, bones, muscles, tendons and all the organs such as the brain and the heart.

Unfortunately, sources of protein are not equal. All *animal* proteins contain all the essential amino acids that you need for life, including proteins from meat, poultry, fish, shellfish, eggs and dairy products. Most vegetable proteins contain most of the essential amino acids but not all. The exception is soya products (such as tofu), which are the only vegetable protein sources that *do* contain all the essential amino acids; if soya-based products are included in reasonable amounts in the diet you can obtain all the essentials that you require. If not, it is necessary to include some source of animal protein in your diet or take a supplement.

Vitamins

Vitamins are required in small quantities to permit certain chemical reactions in all our cells to occur. Although you need the vitamins in tiny quantities, without them (*vitamin deficiency*) you will become seriously unwell. Much more importantly, they are also essential as antioxidants to remove free radicals from the body (see later), a process that prevents disease and ageing. Vitamins are present in high quantities in meat products and fresh vegetables, and virtually not at all in most processed foods. The sources of vitamins are as follows:

Vitamin A

Vitamin A has antioxidant properties effective in maintaining health and slowing the ageing process, and is also essential for our peripheral vision and vision under poor illumination. It acts by facilitating different chemical reactions in every cell of the body, as do many vitamins.

Vitamin A is typically found in plant products with a red pigment such as carrots, red peppers and tomatoes, but is also present in reasonable quantity in both spinach and mangetout. Other foods that contain vitamin A include fish, eggs yolks and dairy products.

Vitamin B_1 (thiamine)

Similarly, vitamin B_1 is an essential factor in most of the chemical reactions, releasing energy from proteins, fats and carbohydrates in every cell in the body. Thiamine is prevalent in nuts and seeds such as cashew nuts, peanuts, Brazil nuts, pine nuts and sesame seeds. Animal sources include salmon and pork.

Vitamin B_2 (riboflavin)

Vitamin B_2, like vitamin B_1, permits the release of energy in every cell in the body, and it is also required for the health of the eyes, the skin and the nervous system. Vitamin B_2 is present in dairy products, poultry, fish, eggs and shellfish, and the plant world supplies B_2 from avocados, mushrooms and almonds.

Vitamin B_3 (niacin)

Similar to many other vitamins, this permits the conversion of food to energy in the cells. Niacin requirements are supplied by fresh meat, chicken and eggs, and particularly high levels are present in fish, particularly salmon and tuna. B_3 is not common in plant products.

Vitamin B_6 (pyridoxine)

Vitamin B_6 is essential for the conversion of amino acids to energy in all of the cells. It is present in pork, tuna, chicken and liver. The plant world supplies B_6 from tomatoes and tomato products, avocados and nuts, such as cashew nuts and walnuts.

Vitamin B_{12} (cyanocobalamin)

B_{12} acts with folate in the production of our genetic material (DNA) and also is particularly important in the development of red blood cells. It is present only in animal products. There has been no vitamin B_{12} discovered in any plant source. It has particularly high concentrations in fish (such as salmon and sardines), liver, eggs and meat.

Folate

Folate reacts in the cells to manufacture the DNA and the building blocks of proteins, the amino acids. It is not common in sources of animal origin, with the exception of liver and kidneys, but is primarily present in vegetable sources (beetroot, asparagus and spinach), wholegrains, nuts (cashews, hazelnuts and peanuts), sunflower seeds and fruits (melons, strawberries, oranges and blackberries).

Vitamin C

Vitamin C functions within the cells of the body to allow chemical reactions to occur, and is particularly important in the formulation of connective tissue such as collagen in blood capillaries, bones, gums and teeth. It is essential for the blood to clot and for nervous function. However, one of its most essential functions is as a major antioxidant to prevent free-radical formation.

Vitamin C is almost totally excluded from products of animal origin, although there is some present in liver and kidneys. Vitamin C is sourced from fruit (such as citrus fruits and strawberries) and vegetables (many green vegetables such as mangetout, but also red and green peppers, tomatoes and broccoli).

Vitamin D

Vitamin D allows the body to absorb calcium, which is essential for nerve and muscle function, particularly that of the heart, and also the formation of bones. Your body can actually make vitamin D via the skin and sunlight. But, as sunlight is not a major component of the climate in the northern hemisphere this is not the best source. Vitamin D is sourced from oily fish (a source of omega-3 fatty acids) such as herring, mackerel, salmon, tuna and sardines. There is a lesser amount of vitamin D in butter and eggs.

Vitamin E

Vitamin E is primarily an antioxidant which mops up free radicals, and thereby prevents ageing and increases immunity. By far the highest sources of vitamin E are avocados, nuts (particularly hazelnuts and almonds), olives and tomatoes, although some lesser amounts are present in fish.

Vitamin K

Vitamin K, like vitamin D, can be produced within the body and is manufactured by some bacteria in the gut. It is essential for making proteins which assist the blood to clot. It comes mainly from the plant world and particularly green vegetables such as broccoli, cabbage, spring onion and spinach.

Minerals

Minerals are elements that are required in only trace amounts, like vitamins, to facilitate reactions in every cell of the body. As with vitamins, although you only need a very small amount, mineral deficiency leads to serious illness.

- **Calcium** allows functions of the body to work, particularly the formation of the skeleton and bones, regulation of the nervous system, and heart-muscle function. It is essential for strong bones, and sourced from dairy products and oily fish (herrings, mackerel, sardines, tuna and salmon), but also from green vegetables (such as parsley and broccoli) and herbs.

- **Chromium** is essential for regulating insulin and therefore both fat metabolism and glucose metabolism. It is present in highest quantities in freshly ground black pepper.

- **Copper** is needed for the absorption of iron and therefore essential to prevent iron-deficiency anaemia. It also is associated with folate in the production of nerve tissue. Copper is sourced especially in the plant world from green vegetables, mushrooms and nuts.

- **Iodine** is essential for the function of the thyroid gland, which controls the speed of our metabolism. It is present in foods of marine origin, such as fish, shellfish and seaweed.

- The most important function of **iron** is in the production of red blood cells, in which it is essential in the transport of oxygen to the tissues. Iron is found in meat, liver, fish and chicken, and the plant world supplies iron from green vegetables, sesame seeds and nuts.

- **Manganese** is particularly needed to produce cholesterol, and utilise body fats. It also has an essential role in the metabolism of sugar in the body. Manganese is present in eggs, green vegetables and nuts.

- **Phosphorus** allows vitamins B_2 and B_3 to be absorbed from the intestine, and it is essential in the formation of bones. It also plays a vital role in the breakdown of body fat and is an important mineral in controlling weight. It is present in seeds (sesame and sunflower), wheatgerm, nuts (cashews, Brazils and pine nuts), eggs, cheese, poultry and liver.

- **Potassium**, with sodium, regulates the transfer of fluid between cells and is also essential in muscle and heart-muscle function. Potassium is present in fish, but again the plant world reigns supreme, with herbs, onions, garlic, vegetables, mushrooms and citrus fruit as sources.

- **Selenium** is a particularly important antioxidant, removing free radicals and preventing cell damage and ageing. Selenium is present in fish, but plant sources include onions, broccoli, tomatoes and bean sprouts.

- **Sodium** is an element that acts in combination with potassium by regulating the fluid across cell membranes. It is essential for the function of the heart and nervous system. It is mainly sourced from meats (especially pork), prawns, smoked salmon and eggs, with a particularly high concentration in tomatoes as a plant source.

- **Sulphur** is a part of insulin and therefore is essential for carbohydrate, protein and fat metabolism. It is also present in many of our structural proteins such as nails, skin and hair. Sulphur is sourced from fish and eggs, but particularly from garlic, onions, cabbage and nuts.

- **Zinc**, too, is a component of insulin, and therefore is essential in the metabolism of proteins, fats and carbohydrates. It is also essential for the immune system. Zinc is present in eggs, but the main source is vegetables, seeds (especially sesame) herbs and nuts such as almonds and cashew nuts.

Free radicals and antioxidants – the key to health

Free radicals and *antioxidants* are common words in health today – but what do the terms actually mean? In every cell of the body (there are up to 50 trillion) there are thousands of chemical reactions occurring every second of every day. During these processes, molecules lose electrons (see below) and become 'free radicals'.

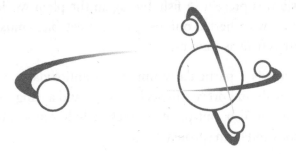

The response of these millions of free radicals is to 'steal' the missing electrons from other molecules (see opposite, top). Unfortunately, this process of 'stealing' electrons weakens the body's defence and immunity mechanisms for infection, even cancer, so the solution is to provide the free radicals with their missing electrons *before* they can cause problems – and this is the function of antioxidants. They provide the missing electrons to the free radicals, thereby negating their damaging properties and solving a very dangerous problem.

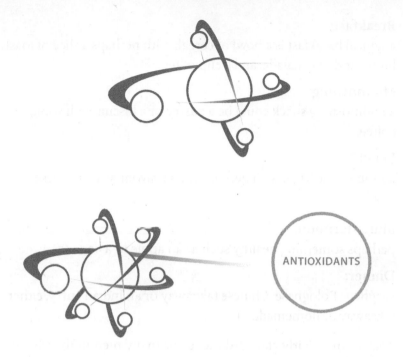

**ANTIOXIDANTS DONATE
ELECTRONS TO FREE RADICAL**

And what is the source of these wondrous, life-saving anti-oxidants? Diet, of course. The naturally occurring antioxidants are found in foods rich in vitamins A, C and E – such as carrots, tomatoes, peppers, green leafy veggies, citrus fruits and avocados – and the mineral selenium.

How to achieve a truly 'healthy' lifestyle

Now that we've explained all the health benefits of changing your lifestyle, the next step is to describe how this can be achieved. Before we do this, let's look at a typical day and see how it compares with our healthy alternative.

Breakfast:
a typical breakfast is a bowl of cereal, with perhaps a slice of toast, butter and marmalade, and a cup of tea.

Midmorning:
a midmorning snack could be a pastry or a biscuit with some coffee.

Lunch:
a simple sandwich, with perhaps tuna mayonnaise or cheese salad.

Mid-afternoon:
perhaps something healthy such as an apple or a banana.

Dinner:
spaghetti Bolognese, Chinese takeaway or an Indian curry, either takeaway or homemade.

That seems a fairly standard menu for many men in their forties, but let's look at just exactly what you are eating here. The above day's consumption makes up about 330 grams of carbohydrates, which is the equivalent of *66 teaspoons of sugar*. That's right, 66 teaspoons of sugar. It is the equivalent of looking at a plate with 66 teaspoons of sugar and eating it. You wouldn't do that, so why do it in another way? But how can this be? There is very little sugar in the food (apart from perhaps the pastry), so where did it come from? Let's look at the facts:

	Carbohydrate
Breakfast	
bowl of cereal	30 g
slice of toast with marmalade	40 g
Midmorning snack	
pastry	40 g
Lunch	
sandwich (bread)	50 g

Afternoon snack

apple   20 g

Dinner

pasta (in spaghetti Bolognese)   75 g

rice (in Chinese or curry meal)   75 g

TOTAL 330 g

A teaspoon of sugar is about 5 grams, so 330 grams of carbohydrates equates to about 66 teaspoons of sugar. But, if you look at what you are eating, it is actually very, very simple to reduce that figure to virtually zero with just a few simple changes. Let's look at an alternative day.

Breakfast

Scrambled eggs with bacon   0 g

Mid-morning snack

not necessary as a breakfast based on protein will release energy gradually and satisfy hunger for hours

Lunch

steak with salad   0 g

or

tuna mayonnaise with salad   0 g

or

chicken mayonnaise with salad   0 g

Mid-afternoon snack

not necessary as protein-based lunch releases energy slowly

Dinner

meat Bolognese with vegetables   10 g

or

Chinese chicken with vegetables   5 g or 10 g

or

Rogan josh curry with vegetables   10 g

TOTAL 10 g

So you can see at a stroke that you can reduce your refined carbo-hydrate intake from 50 teaspoons of sugar to 2 teaspoons of sugar without hunger or denying yourself any good food at all. In fact, the very opposite has occurred, because you are actively eating much more healthy, nutritious and delicious food than previously. The thing to remember is that bread, pasta and rice are merely fillers; they don't actually provide any form of nutrition at all, but merely fill you up with food that is going to make you fat.

Breakfast – the basis of a healthy diet

But how can you possibly produce a healthy breakfast. There is never any time at breakfast. Actually, there is plenty of time, as you are about to realise. A healthy breakfast – which you will enjoy much more than the quick bowl of cereal and slice of toast – is actually very simple to prepare within the normal time con-straints in the morning. It takes almost as much time to pop an egg into a pan, add water and place it on the cooker as it does to pour a bowl of cereal. You can be getting on with other things while it boils.

It merely takes a little planning. We are so accustomed to simply pouring some cereal from a box and quickly wolfing it down that the poor nutritional effects on our body don't seem to matter when we are rushing in the morning. But this doesn't need to be the case.

Let's briefly consider how easy it is to have a healthy nutritious breakfast, which will lower your cholesterol levels, lower your risk of heart disease and give you much more energy throughout the day, in just a few minutes in the morning. The secret is to have food in the fridge and also, if you want to be really quick, use a microwave.

For example, poached eggs can be cooked in a microwave in less than ninety seconds, as can scrambled eggs. Simply mix these with some chopped tomato and cheese and perhaps a few herb leaves (which can be sitting in the kitchen just waiting for you) and you have a delicious breakfast in less than two minutes, which will sustain you throughout the morning. You can also grill bacon or ham, or put them in the microwave.

But this programme is not intended to be proscriptive. If you need to exclude *all* refined carbs *all* of the time, it simply won't be successful, because very few of us have the cast-iron willpower, or the lifestyle, to make this possible. And the most difficult time of day to avoid bread is undoubtedly breakfast. So, if you need to have a slice of toast with your breakfast eggs, do so. To place this in perspective, you are really aiming for a refined-carb content on this programme of no more than 50 grams per day; a 'regular' slice of bread is 18 grams and a small slice only 10 grams, so you have not blown the day by a slice of toast at breakfast. We have even given the option of toast with eggs, cheese and mushrooms for breakfast in Appendix A – but avoid them if you can, and definitely no bread for the first two weeks.

Continental-style breakfasts with cheese, meats, ham, chicken and perhaps some Continental hams such as pastrami or chorizo are all available to protect your heart. This may seem like heresy given the content of saturated fats in pastrami and chorizo, but bear in mind that the source of 85 per cent of all fats in your blood originate from your liver – not your diet – and they are produced in the liver *as a direct consequence of the insulin response to carbohydrates in the diet, not fats.*

When you are really in a hurry, the simplest way is to have a Continental breakfast, obviously without croissant, jam or pastries. These are the sorts of delicious foods that can be included:

Cheese

All cheeses are suitable for this, and remember that cheese does not actually increase your cholesterol level. So you can enjoy any of the delicious cheeses available such as Emmental, Jarlsberg, Brie, Mozzarella, Gouda, Edam . . . the list is almost endless.

Continental meats

Continental meats are ideal for this purpose, as they have virtually no refined carbohydrates whatsoever. And nothing could be quicker. Take beef, for instance. Beef is a no-carbohydrate food that is absolutely delicious either cold or hot. This can easily be picked up from the deli or supermarket as smoked, salted or pastrami.

Poultry

What could be better than some delicious cooked chicken or turkey for breakfast?

Eggs

In any form. Simply, for this type of breakfast, hard-boil an egg for six minutes and enjoy it with the rest of the meal.

Fish

Don't forget fish as an important source of protein for breakfast. You don't even need to cook it just buy some precooked fish (such as trout, kippers or mackerel) and have it either cold or heated up in the microwave for thirty seconds.

So you can see that having a non-carbohydrate breakfast is not that difficult, and protects your heart. But you don't need to actually cook or even prepare your own breakfast. There are probably many outlets on the way to work where you can have a cooked breakfast of bacon and eggs, which again will protect your heart and allow you to lose weight at the same time.

The real health hazards of 'fast foods'

So-called 'fast' foods have virtually destroyed our normal way of living, and have certainly destroyed our health. Let's look at how these fast foods affect your blood sugar levels, and your ability to work throughout the day.

Remember that fast foods are basically full of refined carbohydrates and trans fats, the very foods that are guaranteed to make you unhealthy and fat, and have heart disease. When you have a high-carb breakfast, such as cereal or toast, your blood sugar rises, then insulin kicks in and lowers it once again so that by mid morning you have a low blood sugar and you're hungry. So you have to have more sugar, and so you naturally take a pastry or a biscuit, and once again it raises your sugar level but again you get this big hit of insulin, which is there to lower sugar, and by lunchtime your blood sugar is low again.

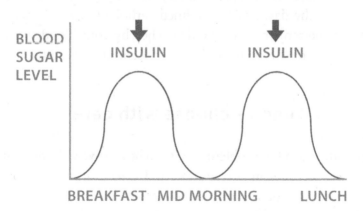

Once again, after the sandwich with its 50 grams of carbohydrate (or 8–10 teaspoons of sugar), your blood sugar rises and falls again by mid afternoon and so the inevitable piece of fruit or biscuit is absolutely essential because you are hungry.

And this pattern is repeated day after day with various episodes of raised blood sugar at the peaks and low blood sugar at the troughs. You literally cannot possibly avoid sugary foods, because the insulin cycle is driving you to eat more.

It is much worse than just a cycle of hunger and eating, however. During the periods when your blood sugar is low, during the troughs, you start to experience the typical symptoms of low blood sugar (not surprisingly), which are:

- reduced concentration
- irritability
- low mood
- possibly sweating
- hunger pangs

These are all symptoms that we are sure you have experienced on a daily basis for a very long time. Simply having a substantial breakfast will solve this problem. By having a good breakfast at the start of the day, avoiding refined carbohydrates, you set the scene for the remainder of the day, whereby your blood sugar is stable, your mood is better and your concentration is better.

Lunch – choose with care

Lunch can be a major problem – or it can be relatively simple. Once again, the secret is in preparation and organisation, and being determined that you're not going to put on weight.

Most choices for lunch are just simply complicated ways of making you fat. Almost all convenience foods are highly fattening, and have a distinct predilection to produce heart disease, diabetes, weakness and fatigue. But it is certainly not all doom and gloom.

In general, most men aged over forty have lives governed by

convenience foods and family attitudes. Convenience and portability are the common threads, and products that offer this are most likely to appeal to men in their forties. Manufacturers have encouraged this idea because most convenience foods, particularly at lunchtime, are cheap and easy to produce, with high profit margins, and are purchased by men who have busy lives and don't have time to have a proper meal. For example, panini, ciabatta, call it what you will, is nothing more than 80 per cent bread and 20 per cent nutrition. As bread costs virtually nothing, the typical sandwich has a huge profit margin.

Lunch falls into two main categories for the busy professional:

- takeaway lunch (or occasionally prepared at home and taken to the office)

- restaurant meal

For the majority of men in their forties and fifties, a takeaway lunch is the only option available in a busy lifestyle, but it can still be part of a healthy lifestyle geared to reducing the risk of heart disease and improving health, by following a few simple rules.

Of course, the programme becomes less restricted as it develops, but it is essential to get your body back into gear as quickly as possible. It's probably best to outline those foods to be *avoided* for lunch – as this group constitutes the most common male choices.

Foods to be avoided at lunchtime are:

- Pizza. The base of a pizza is about 73 per cent carbohydrate, so a typical pizza may have as much as 120 grams of carbs (24 teaspoons of sugar).

- Noodles and pasta. As always, most pasta is about 70–75 per cent carbs.

- Processed foods. These include pasties, pies and sausage rolls.

- Potato crisps.

- All breads. This category includes panini, baguettes, bagels, tortillas, bread, rolls. These are the staple diet at lunchtime and usually contain 30–50 grams of carbs per sandwich (6–10 teaspoons of sugar).

■ Cakes, pastries and chocolates.

And of course most takeaway foods have to be avoided on this sort of programme, as most are very high in carbs:

■ Burgers. Almost all burgers have a bun, which contains about 60 grams of carbs, or about 10–12 teaspoons of sugar.

■ Fried chicken. Fried chicken of course is perfectly healthy. However, the batter around it is most certainly not and must be avoided.

■ Chips.

■ Jacket potatoes.

■ Chinese takeaway. Actually, most Chinese takeaway is low-GI if you avoid the rice, but unfortunately it often contains a lot of MSG, and that makes it unhealthy.

■ Indian takeaway. Once again, the basis of Indian takeaway is very healthy, but the rice, naan bread and chapatti are incredibly high in carbs, and therefore incredibly high in sugar.

This doesn't seem to leave many appetising – and available – lunch options, but nothing could be further from the truth.

Really healthy lunch options

Salad

This is not the typical salad of a few green leaves and tomatoes and nothing else. This is *man* salad, with beef, chicken, tuna, smoked salmon and lashings of mayonnaise.

This type of salad ensures that you won't be hungry for hours and your blood-sugar levels will stabilise. And, as an added incentive, cholesterol will be reduced. The old-fashioned idea of a skimpy salad, with virtually nothing in it, being healthy, is obviously incorrect. If you eat much less than you need, you are bound to become malnourished. It is simply not possible to take in all the vitamins and minerals you need on some form of starvation diet.

On the other hand, if we recall that it is not the *amount* of food that you eat for health, but rather the *type* of food, this comes into its own with lunch. Let's just briefly examine all of the different types of food that you can enjoy with a substantial salad at lunchtime:

- tiger prawns
- ham and mustard
- cheese
- roast beef
- egg mayonnaise or boiled eggs
- avocado
- chargrilled peppers
- chicken (in any form)
- bacon, lettuce and tomato
- coronation chicken
- salmon
- chicken and bacon
- prawn with mayo
- chicken tikka
- tuna mayo
- roast pork
- cheese with pancetta

- ploughman's with cheese of any form, onions and pickle

- smoked turkey with cranberry sauce

- mozzarella with tomato

- olives

- herrings

- taramasalata

- sun-dried tomatoes

- artichokes

- tzatziki

- cold meats, such as hams or salami

- cabanas

As you can see, the choice from your local deli is almost limitless. Provided you avoid the breads, almost all the foods in your local delicatessen are suitable for a healthy, weight-reducing, heart-protective programme. And, if you don't have a local delicatessen, try your local supermarket, which almost certainly sells most of these foods. If you do have a local deli, get them to make up a large salad box with substantial fillings on which you cannot possibly be hungry for most of the afternoon.

This doesn't take much time. It may not take any longer to walk to the local deli than the local hamburger outlet. And of course, it is essential that you add healthy fats in with your lunch in order that it is absorbed slowly and provides energy all afternoon. So add in such fats as extra-virgin olive oil, dressings or mayonnaise with your lunch because, as we have seen, these types of fat are not the ones that cause raised cholesterol: on the contrary, they actually help to lower cholesterol.

What could be less restrictive than a programme with all of these foods to make you healthy and lose weight at the same time?

Restaurant lunches

Of course, if you intend to go to a restaurant, then simply follow the rules on page 175 and there won't be a problem. Avoid bread, rice, pasta, potatoes (in any form) and sweet foods, and the choice is yours. This means that any form of meat or poultry with vegetables, or fish, shellfish and delicious sauces in almost any combination are safe, healthy and heart-friendly.

Really healthy dinner options

Dinner is definitely much easier than lunch, because the working day is usually over and you are in control. The secret, as in all of these meals, is preparation.

Keep a checklist in the back of your mind as to what you can and cannot eat, according to the schedule in Chapter 1 (see 'High-GI foods' on page 9), and you really can't go wrong. It means that the choice is immense. Of course, the selections of different meats, fish, shellfish and poultry, with vegetables in virtually any format, cover a very broad area, but listed below are many of the various combinations that you can have to demonstrate the huge variety available.

These recipes and more are all included in Appendix A. They are easy to prepare and taste absolutely delicious – and obviously negate the myth that 'healthy' food is boring. And, of course, these are only a small selection of delicious meals that can be easily made from the ingredients included in the diet; the potential is limited only by your imagination.

- Chargrilled Tuna Steaks with Oriental Dressing
- Chargrilled Chicken with Chilli Salsa
- Crunchy Cod Fillets with Herb Salad
- Citrus Scallops

- Cooked Tiger Prawns with Seasonal Mixed Fruit

- Fresh Mussel Salad with Aromatic Ginger Dressing

- Green Apple and Roquefort Omelette

- Grilled Asparagus with Italian-style Sauce

- Mexican Scrambled Eggs

- Moroccan Lamb

- Oven-baked Duck with Tarragon Dressing

- Oven-baked Ricotta with Vine-ripened Cherry Tomatoes

- Pan-fried Steak with Baked Halloumi

- Poached Chicken with Robust Red Wine

- Roasted Veggie Fusion

- Smoked Salmon Sashimi

- Spicy Venison with Coriander Salad

- Stir-fried Tiger Prawns with Chilli Mixed Peppers

- Walnut, Herb and Vegetable Medley

- White Sole Fillets with Herb Dressing

Restaurant dinners

Of course, it is even easier to eat out than to prepare food yourself. The choice is almost limitless, and all you have to do is to avoid the obvious exclusion areas, and stick with the huge remainder. For example, in an Italian restaurant avoid the pizza and pasta, and start perhaps with some scallops Venetian style or prosciutto and melon and follow with perhaps some poached salmon with vegetables.

In a Chinese restaurant stick with meat or fish or shellfish with vegetables and simply avoid the rice.

In an Indian restaurant, once again stick with the meat, fish and shellfish recipes, avoiding all rice and breads such as naan, chapatti and poppadoms.

Thai restaurants are even easier because all you have to do is avoid the rice and most of the remainder of the dishes are healthy.

However, that said, the freshest food is always that prepared at home, or bought ready prepared for home use, and in the first month of the programme this is by far the healthiest and most effective way of arresting any problems for your heart and accelerating health-giving properties.

Planning

The secret of a successful programme is planning. This means being prepared for the various circumstances that will arise unexpectedly. However, initially, the most important task is to maintain a well-stocked larder. The problem really stems from the fact that there is very little time in modern life. Everyone is busy and the casualty is usually healthy meals. If you keep a stock of certain basic essential foods constantly available, the temptation to snack on *unhealthy* foods or have a quick fast meal by way of an oven-ready pizza will simply disappear. As we have seen, it is very simple to have quick, healthy – and fast – meals without resorting to pizza or its equivalent. The essential ingredients are relatively simple, but cover most situations very well:

- black peppercorns
- butter
- cheese
- citrus fruits
- crème fraîche
- extra-virgin olive oil

- free-range eggs

- fresh fish

- fresh ginger root

- fresh poultry

- fresh tomatoes

- fresh vegetables, especially spring onions, broccoli and peppers

- garlic

- herbs

- mayonnaise

- mustard (according to taste)

- nuts, especially walnuts, hazelnuts and Brazils

- onions

- prawns

- sea salt

- shellfish

- tinned tomatoes

- tinned tuna

- tomato purée

If you keep the larder stocked up, and replenish it weekly with these ingredients, you will always be able to have quick and delicious meals at short notice without reaching for the next refined carb.

Read the label

Although this programme is based primarily on fresh food, obviously it becomes necessary to use pre-prepared foods on occasions. However, the golden rule is that you must always read the label to determine what the package actually contains. Many foods contain hidden sugars, often labelled as 'carbohydrate', and, as you are now aware, carbohydrate is just another word for sugar because carbohydrates are simply sugar molecules joined together.

The nutritional content is displayed on the label of every packaged food and is usually in the following format:

Typical values	Nutrition per 100g	Per pack
Energy	420 kJ	1,480 kJ
	102 kcal	351 kcal
Protein	10.9 g	38.2 g
Carbohydrate	4.2 g	15.1 g
of which sugars	1.9 g	7.6 g
Fat	5.4 g	19.1 g
of which saturates	0.7 g	2.8 g
Fibre	1.2 g	4.4 g
Sodium	0.41 g	1.32 g
Equivalent of salt	1.1 g	3.4 g

This is much simpler than it seems. Always read the carbohydrate value, as this provides the *actual* total sugar value. Don't be mislead by the statement 'of which sugars'. This is designed to cause confusion. Manufacturers tend to make it clear that the sugars to which they refer are actually white sugar. So, for example, a typical pasta would have 73 grams of carbohydrate per 100 grams (73 per cent), of which the sugar is 0 grams. In actual fact, it should read 'of which sugar is 73 grams', because the carbohydrate will entirely convert to sugar, just not the white sugar that we call sucrose. So look at the carbohydrate content rather than the sugar content, and just read that as actual sugar. Anything greater than 7–8 grams per 100 (7–8 per cent) is probably going to be too high, so avoid those foods.

The dangerous hours

Planning what you eat is as important as every other aspect of a healthy lifestyle, in fact probably more so, because you literally are what you eat. However, this is one area where we tend to neglect our responsibilities and consider food more as merely a fuel or energy source and little else. Food should, of course, encompass all of the nutrition we need to be active and healthy, not be just a source (in many instances) of empty calories that provide no function. As with any successful operation, you need to plan ahead. As we have already seen, the first and single most important thing is to ensure you have the food in the kitchen that you will need, because that prevents the snacking problem. As a corollary, you also want to remove from your kitchen the food that you don't want, so empty the fridge and get rid of all of the convenience foods that are high in refined carbohydrates that you don't need and don't want. But, in addition, you need to have a plan in place for the many occasions where unexpected events occur. This is what we call 'the dangerous hours': those times when you just cannot have a smoked-salmon salad.

It is remarkably simple to plan for virtually every situation by programming your body using specific eating and behavioural techniques.

So when are 'the dangerous hours'? See the clocks opposite.

The main reason we eat at odd times such as these is that we haven't had an adequate meal at normal times. In other words, if you have a healthy breakfast then your blood sugar will simply not reduce by 11 a.m. and you won't need to snack. The problem,

| 11AM | 4PM | 7PM | 10PM |

of course, is the word *healthy*. Healthy breakfast is promoted as being a cereal with (usually) skimmed milk, followed by croissant and jam, and this is absolutely guaranteed to lower your blood sugar by 10.30 and set you reaching for the morning muffin. Let's reiterate what we stated earlier (see page 173): breakfast of cereal and toast elevates the blood sugar initially. But by 10.30 the insulin response has been stimulated and the blood sugar has dropped dramatically until it reaches very low levels, the condition known as *hypoglycaemia*.

At this stage it is essential for you to have that midmorning snack, and that muffin becomes irresistible. Of course many offices make the situation worse by actually providing muffins and pastries, or handy vending machines full of sugary snacks. If, on the other hand, you have a couple of poached eggs (with a single slice of toast as part of your daily carb intake) in the morning, your blood sugar elevates but does not dip at 10.30, and you will have energy until lunchtime and beyond. The problem is solved simply by planning.

However, coffee breaks are used either as a necessary break from work or simply an occasion for socialising, and most men give little thought to the importance of what they eat or drink during these unguarded moments. So, let's first assess likely patterns of behaviour, then form a plan of action.

Drinks

The air in modern offices is normally dry, which increases the need for rehydration. Water coolers are often underused except in the height of summer. However, dehydration is a major cause of poor performance.

Fizzy drinks provide an immediate caffeine buzz with the added disadvantage of a multitude of undesirable chemicals: artificial sweeteners, colorants, additives and so forth. Opting for the stimulation of coffee is fine as long as you are aware that coffee increases dehydration. The same is true of tea, although to a much lesser degree. So match each cup of coffee or tea with a glass of water for improved performance and health.

We'll continue to explore the dangerous hours in the following sections.

The ubiquitous effects of food

Food alters bodily shape, our social life, our moods, our chances of meeting the right partner and the quality and length of our lives.

The body needs food to function and gives signals when more fuel is required. As with every other bodily need, attitudes to food vary from indifferent to obsessive; in a similar manner, the body's signalling system ranges from inefficient to hyperactive. As with all body functions, it has been and is shaped by our past experiences and current actions.

It is necessary to become food-aware. Do you know that foods such as porridge – which is a less-refined carb, so has lower GI – are not only more satisfying but also increase the brain's level of serotonin, the feel-good chemical?

Similarly, in the afternoon, a higher-carb lunch results in low blood sugar by 3.30–4 p.m., prompting you to look for the inevitable sugar top-up. It is a simple physiological problem: you have low blood sugar so your body craves sugar. While it can sometimes be difficult to ensure a good lunch every day, based mainly on protein and salad or vegetables, the secret to preventing the late-afternoon 'dangerous hour' is to prepare in advance. Snacks that can be enjoyed at this time include nuts, seeds or (for the more adventurous) a little smoked salmon. Most offices have an office fridge and you can keep some smoked salmon, chicken or tuna mayonnaise in it, all of which are easily available from your local delicatessen or supermarket. These foods are particularly effective at satisfying hunger immediately and stabilising your blood-sugar requirements for hours.

Where is your mind/brain in this cycle of self-destruction? Thoughtless choices dictated by habit and poor food decisions are affecting your performance at work, the shape of your body and the quality of your relationships.

The tea-trolley temptation

> 'I can resist anything except temptation'
>
> – OSCAR WILDE, *Lady Windermere's Fan*

To avoid all the temptations in offices and workplaces, take your own healthy snacks, or buy them from the local delicatessen, and the craving for sugar will disappear. Avoiding fast food and eating for health is a balance between:

- the need to eat
- constraints on time
- options available
- choices made

Use job skills to regain control of this essential part of your life. Habit shapes behaviour and choices. The first step is role reversal: take charge of your eating rather than let poor food choices control you.

The need to eat

The need is to restore physical energy and mental resilience in order to perform at a level that is satisfying and productive. The eating patterns of high-performance sportsmen are designed to deliver sustained energy in some sports, and short bursts of energy in others. Nutrition is as important as every other aspect of their training programme and, indeed, is its central component. All such programmes are built on a solid base of healthy foods, with a well-designed balance of all of the essential nutrients to ensure optimal performance.

There should be no difference between the world-class athlete and everyone else. If such attention to nutrition is taken by people who perform under optimal conditions as an absolute require-ment of their chosen occupation, the same attention to the detail of nutrition should be taken by everyone – especially as you are required to perform daily in less-than-ideal situations, not only at work but also at home.

Constraints of time

During recession, men tend to remain longer at the office. Research shows that one in four men skips the lunch break completely. Ten per cent take less than twenty minutes while the average lunch break lasts thirty-five minutes. The shorter the break, the more important to utilise it effectively. Remember the logic of 'rubbish in produces rubbish out'. Planning is the key to successful nutri-tion – and therefore health. Whatever the length, use the lunch break to boost mental activity and restore physical energy.

Options available

In Western society, few have ever experienced real hunger. Food choices are based on what you want, not on what you can get or need. Usually men in the work environment unthinkingly meet their wants but not their needs. Wants are basic responses to sights and smells based on habit and familiarity – and the drive to con-sume unhealthy refined carbs due to the unacceptably high insulin levels produced by the typical Western diet.

Developing a healthy relationship with food has only positives:

used efficiently, food is fuel for the body, allows the mind to function optimally, plays an important role in social relations, gives pleasurable sensations of taste and the enjoyment of shared social occasions.

Choices made

For many men, the choice between high-carb foods (such as pastries and biscuits) and low-carb alternatives (dips and nuts) is a lost cause. But the former is really nursery food, ideal for growing, active children, rich in carbohydrates, which they burn off in games. Are you still at the nursery food stage?

Supermarket bread counters and fast food outlets rely on smell to stimulate customers to want and then buy what they may not need. If your colleagues are consuming fast foods it takes considerable willpower to be different.

An abundance of low-carb, low-GI foods are available. Read the labels carefully. Heart disease, diabetes and hypertension are the well-established physical effects of a high-carb diet, but these foods also have detrimental effects on mental health: Spanish scientists have found a link between eating junk food containing harmful trans fats and an increased risk of depression. These fats are found in fast foods, pastries, cakes and biscuits. But olive oil and healthier polyunsaturated fats appear to have the opposite effect, helping to keep people cheerful.

After-work temptations

The next danger period occurs at about 6.30–7 p.m., when you return from work famished and stretch for the crisps or crackers. Once again, the secret is planning. Make sure you have nuts or, better still, dips and crudités available. We have a section later that explains how dips can be made simply, or they can be purchased (always read the label to make sure that you are not buying too much sugar inadvertently). Humus, tzatziki, raita and guacamole are all excellent combined with celery, carrot, broccoli and cauli-flower crudités. Problem solved.

The final problem of the day is usually before bed, but once again this is solved by ensuring that dinner is designed to release blood sugars at an even rate. So, if you have, for example, curry with rice, the rice makes up about 120–130 grams of carbohydrate (26 teaspoons of sugar) and this once again elevates your blood sugar and then drops it dramatically, so that you are hungry again in the latter part of the evening. By simply exchanging the rice for vegetables, you'll ensure that the blood sugar remains stable and the pre-bed hunger pangs simply don't occur. It is important to realise that spices in curry are among the healthiest foods on the planet. Spices have the highest concentration of antioxidants of any food and it is not the curry that is the problem but the naan bread, the chapattis and the rice that accompany it. So simply exclude those and the problem is solved once again.

One of the most important aspects of a low-carb programme is the realisation that it is self-fulfilling: as your insulin level reduces, your desire to consume these sugary foods reduces with it and the problem of snacking simply disappears. There is no will-power required: quite simply your desire to eat those types of food disappears.

It is important to recognise that the 'dangerous hours' exist and to develop coping strategies to deal with them *before the problem arises*. Once the problem has arisen and you have no appropriate food or coping strategy in place, it is too late. Your blood sugar is low, you need to eat, and there is nothing healthy available. If, on the other hand, you have prepared beforehand by either eating appropriately at mealtimes or by having healthy snacks available to tide you over the problem, there is no problem.

Often you may feel that there is simply no time to cook when you arrive home late from work. However, *there is always time to cook, particularly if cooking can be almost as quick as heating up a take-away*. Once again, the solution lies in preparation and the realisation that 'fast' food does not need to be unhealthy food. We have provided a number of very simple recipes in Appendix A, which can be prepared in minutes, are healthy and delicious, and prevent you having health problems in the future.

Keep track of what you eat

As a final tip, keep a food diary. Set up a spreadsheet on your computer, or buy a small notebook, and record everything that you consume. This is both cathartic, as it encourages you to be careful, and shows you how simple things can creep into your diet on a regular basis without your realising.

It doesn't seem to matter if you have the odd extra slice of toast, but when that adds to the odd piece of chocolate and the occasional piece of cake in a day you can suddenly see how sometimes 'odd' little inconsistencies become very significant indeed. So take the time to keep that food diary – it's amazing how effective it is in helping you adhere to the programme.

SUMMARY

▶ 'Real food' is something that you can consume for nutrition, which is alive or was alive until recently, and which has not been artificially modified by man.

▶ Food consists of six categories: carbohydrates, protein, fat, vitamins, minerals and, most important of all, water.

▶ All of the above are essential for health except carbohydrates – especially refined carbohydrates.

▶ 'Essential' fatty acids are necessary for health – but must be in the correct proportion, which is 2:1 for

→

omega-6 to omega-3 fatty acids. The current ratio in the Western diet is 20:1 – which is decidedly unhealthy.

▶ Trans fats – present in many processed foods – do not exist in nature and are the really dangerous fats.

▶ All 'essential' amino acids are present only in foods of animal extraction – except soya-based products.

▶ Vitamins and minerals are essential for health, especially the antioxidant vitamins A, C and E, and the mineral selenium, which remove free radicals from the body, thereby slowing the ageing process and improving immunity from infection and cancer.

▶ Reduce your intake of refined carbohydrates to 50 grams per day – or less – for health.

▶ Become food-aware – read the label.

▶ In practice being food-aware also means the following:

　▶ Have a reasonable breakfast, which does not necessarily mean a large breakfast but certainly one that will sustain you throughout the morning. In this regard, eggs are undoubtedly king.

　▶ Make time to have a meal in the middle of the day and later in the evening. Remember, it is your health that is at stake and there is always time.

　▶ Have healthy snacks available for the initial stages of the programme so that, if you do get caught short, you are ready. Within a few weeks, snacking will not be a problem, as your desire to eat these foods will reduce very quickly.

　▶ Manage stress. Stressing causes binge eating and is as important to control as your food intake.

→

▶ Never follow a low-calorie diet. A low-calorie diet is basically starvation, and when you do so your body simply craves food most of the time. Under this circumstance, even with the best preparation, it is absolutely impossible to avoid temptation and so you eat the wrong food, which defeats the whole object (which is primarily health rather than weight loss, although the latter reduces anyway).

▶ Maintain a food diary. Being food-aware means being aware of the food you consume on a daily basis.

11

The Action Plan

Sometimes it is difficult to appreciate fully the extent to which an unhealthy lifestyle has progressed, because it becomes the 'norm' due to the pressures and strains of everyday life. Men are much more likely to be unaware of their stressful lifestyle than women, and of the ways in which their lifestyle is making them unwell. However, the deterioration is usually so insidious that it is often not addressed until it is too late. Having discussed all of the various component parts to a 'new' you, it is time to develop an effective strategy. Obviously, one strategy does not fit all, and so it is important to develop your own plan of action, with different emphases on the various parameters, depending on which need the most attention:

- eat your way to health

- protect your heart

- chill out

- drink up

- posture, posture, posture

- muscle up

However, it's important to realise that, provided you incorporate all of the essential components of the programme, *you will achieve measurable positive results within two weeks*. Of course, you are not going to reverse all of the problems accumulated over many years in this short period, but you will certainly begin to see results in weight reduction and energy very quickly; more importantly, the internal markers for heart disease and diabetes (blood fats, insulin and glucose) show dramatic reductions within two weeks and these are easily sustained.

Eat your way to health

Now you can appreciate that you really are what you eat. By piling into the fast-food carbs, you are literally killing yourself. A diet high in refined carbs, typical of a modern busy lifestyle, is simply a complicated way of ensuring that you develop heart disease, diabetes and stroke. But you can now see how easy it is to avoid the terrible triumvirate with simple alterations to your daily routine.

- **Cut out the bread, pasta and rice** These are merely fillers. Replace them with vegetables and salad. Of course, the initial stage of the programme requires a virtually complete ban on refined carbs: a maximum of one slice of wholemeal bread per day, with no rice or pasta. This is essential as you are reversing a trend that has been developing insidiously, usually for many years. When the programme is established, which varies between individuals but is never less than six weeks, you can gradually introduce a moderate amount of wholegrain rice or pasta on a maximum of two occasions per week. You will know when your insulin levels have reduced sufficiently because you will not physically desire more than this amount. If you do, you need to stay on the initial programme for longer.

■ **Feast on protein** Protein is essential for health. Obviously, in the very rare cases of those who have kidney failure, protein can be dangerous, but presumably, as that affects such a tiny proportion of the population, it is irrelevant in most cases, and anyone who has kidney failure is very sick indeed, so you need have no concerns on that score. For everyone else, protein is healthy – full stop. Most of your body consists of protein, which needs to be constantly replenished, so enjoy protein in your diet.

Remember that fast food does not have to be unhealthy. Smoked salmon, chicken and guacamole can be purchased readymade. The secret is in planning ahead. Planning is essentially the main problem in most lives: we simply don't have time – or don't think we have time – to prepare in advance, but time is there for everyone exactly the same. Remember that time is not tangible: it is merely an intangible which inexorably progresses irrespective of any of our wishes or actions. The secret is in how you use that time, and one of the most important uses is planning your food menu. You are inevitably going to eat at various times during the day, whether you plan or not. The difference is that by planning you can be healthy and, by failing to ensure you have the correct foods available, you will be unhealthy.

Food preparation and cooking

Many people believe that they do not have enough time in their busy life to cook. But by simply planning ahead and organising your time carefully it is perfectly feasible to enjoy healthy food that can also be 'fast'. Quick, nutritious meals can be made simply by buying the right ingredients in advance. Many foods can be ready-cooked (such as chicken, beef, salami or prawns), which is ideal for a hectic schedule.

Even more simply, you can cook these meals very quickly using modern technology: the microwave. Microwave cooking is often thought of as a way of heating up ready-prepared meals. However, it is actually very versatile and can produce virtually all meals quickly with little effort. It requires almost no expertise in cooking whatsoever. For example, place a fillet of salmon on a microwave-safe plate, cook in the microwave oven (850W) on 'high' for 2–3 minutes and it is perfectly cooked and tastes delicious – with hardly any conscious effort.

Let's look at some of the main food groups and see how these can be easily cooked quickly, fitting into even the busiest lifestyle.

Fish and shellfish: the ideal fast food

- Ready prepared. Fish and shellfish come in more varieties of ready-prepared food than any other. You can buy prawns, salmon, smoked trout, herring and mussels, which, when combined with delicious salads or stir-fried vegetables, provide an instant meal in themselves.

- Baking. Useful for fish but not shellfish. Place the fish fillet on a baking tray, dot with butter and transfer to a pre-heated oven (180°C, gas mark 4) for 15–20 minutes and the meal is effortlessly cooking while your time is free.

- Frying. Fish are ideally suited for frying with a little butter or extra-virgin olive oil and, once again, will be ready within five minutes.

- Stir-frying. Shellfish in particular are ideal for stir-frying; when some stir-fried vegetables are added, it is almost an instant meal.

- Steaming. Once again, this is a quick way of cooking fish and shellfish requiring virtually no effort.

■ Grilling. Fish cook very quickly under a hot grill, and once again are ready within 5–6 minutes.

■ Microwaving. Even easier, place the fish in a microwave (850W) and microwave on 'high' for 2–3 minutes while you toss the salad.

Poultry

■ Ready prepared. Pre-cooked chicken or turkey (or any other type of poultry), with or without sauces, once again when combined with stir-fry vegetables or salad, provides the ultimate 'fast' supper.

■ Baking. Place the chicken breast on a baking tray, dot with butter and cook for 15–20 minutes in a preheated oven at 180°C (gas mark 4) for a quick ready meal.

■ Microwaving. Poultry is very amenable to cooking by microwave.

■ Roasting. Of course, if you have time and can plan ahead, placing a chicken or duck in the oven could not be simpler and provides a meal later in the day.

Pork, lamb and beef

Almost unlimited varieties of pre-cooked meats are available from delis and supermarkets. They can range from simple 'pure' cooked meats (roast beef, lamb or pork) to the various salamis, chorizo and pastramis.

■ Grilling. Ideal for larger cuts of meat such as chops and steaks.

■ Frying. Shallow-fat frying, particularly with extra-virgin olive oil or butter, is very healthy and a very quick way of preparing smaller meat cuts.

- Baking. Casseroles take a little time before they are ready (2–3 hours) but, with a little preparation and planning ahead, the meal is simply prepared and well worth the effort.

- Roasting. Again, roasting means planning ahead, but placing beef, pork or lamb in the oven and enjoying the meal a couple of hours later really could not be much simpler.

Vegetables

Fresh vegetables, freshly prepared, are always best, as they retain most of their nutrition. However, in a busy lifestyle this is usually not possible, particularly on weekdays. But, ready-prepared vegetables are widely available as either vegetables themselves or salads. French beans, sugar-snap peas, carrots, broccoli, cauliflower, mangetout and asparagus are available in pre-prepared form for those with very busy lifestyles and just need to be cooked using one of the following techniques – although the preparation time is so short that (and the nutritional content so much higher) that it's probably easier to prepare the veggies yourself.

- Steaming. What could be simpler than placing the vegetables in the steamer, leaving them to cook and returning ten minutes later to a perfectly cooked meal?

- Stir-frying. Stir-fried vegetables retain their nutrition and cook in minutes.

- Microwaving. Once again, microwaving proves an excellent way of cooking, by retaining nutrition and allowing the vegetables to cook without any effort whatsoever.

So eat your way to a better life.

Protect your heart

Although this is probably the most important section on health, it is not an individual entity, because heart protection comes from all of the previous advice combined. So, if you want to protect your heart, you need to eat properly (and that means cutting out refined carbs) and ensure that you have a good positive balance of vitamins and minerals. You need to reduce your stress levels because stress is the ultimate heart killer, and this means making time for yourself and going through some simple exercises taking no more than ten minutes per day. Ten minutes is less than a 120th of your day, so we're sure you can afford less than 1 per cent for heart protection. Again, exercise is free and the time is there.

Follow the simple isometric programme on pages 130–41 to begin the process, or commence the isotonic programme on pages 141–53 – but, if you are a novice to exercise, *take it slowly and gradually to begin: too much exercise too soon is a recipe for disaster*. Even if you don't want to take the time for exercise, walking an extra two stops for the bus and parking your car further away so that you get that 20–30 minutes three times per week is simple and practical – and is free.

Concentrate on the three main aspects of heart disease prevention:

- diet, reducing refined carbohydrates

- reducing stress levels by positive strategies

- exercise

So if you want to have a healthy life, think heart. Many goals seem to be impossible as one ages, when in fact most reasonable health goals, particularly relating to cardiac health, are achievable. Be positive in your attitude and you can make it happen.

Attitude, attitude, attitude

Having discussed these various components, we need now to look at strategies. As I said previously, no one strategy fits all, so it is important for you to take what you like from this and build it into your working day. Try to build up slowly: there is no point in trying to do everything at once.

- **Focus on realistic achievements** Visualise what you want to achieve and when. The easiest way to do this is to close your eyes, visualise how you would like to be, and then develop a strategy to achieve it.

- **Establish the reason** Decide why you want to make these achievements and, until you do, don't start. In other words, there must be a reason if you are going to be successful.

- **Believe in yourself** You can literally do anything within reason – provided you are realistic and are prepared to be patient to achieve your goals.

- **Prioritise** Time is not a tangible: it is an intangible. You can do with it as you wish. 'There is no time' means 'I don't want to make time'. Think of all the wasted time in your day. Sit down and make a table of all of the times that you don't use it (and you will be amazed at how much of the time that is), and then realise that there is time for virtually everything you really want to do.

- **Start now** There is no tomorrow, only now. Without being too melodramatic, tomorrow may not come, and it certainly won't come if you delay action now. So start today, and focus on achieving a few more (realistic) goals every day.

- **Don't be negative** If it does not work on one day, don't beat yourself up about it. If the diet slips on one day, make a resolution to correct it the next. If you miss out an exercise one day, don't necessarily double the exercise the next but just have the resolution to do it. Remember, negativity merely increases stress levels and will reverse your achievements.

It's natural for most of us to view the negative rather than the positive aspects of our lives, but the mantra 'accentuate the positive and eliminate the negative' is the most important approach to attitude. If you have a pessimistic or negative mental attitude, this increases stress levels and predisposes you to illness. It doesn't matter how bad things seem: go back to basics – you are alive, and that is better than the alternative. From that beginning you can achieve almost anything (within reason) and you must approach this with as much resolve you would any physical attribute such as diet or exercise. The human mind has a potential to cause illness that is always underestimated, and a healthy mind is essential to the development of a healthy body.

Chill out

As we have already seen, stress is a major problem for men from their forties onwards. You need to develop a strategy to address this, and make sure the strategy for your mind is at least as important as, if not more than, the strategy for your physical health.

Recognise the signs

This is the single most important factor in combating stress. Unless you recognise the signs, the problem inevitably progresses. As we have already discussed, men are much more likely to be unaware of their stress levels than women. Unexplained headaches, onset of indigestion, reduced sex drive and depression are all early signs, but unfortunately they tend to develop slowly and insidiously. It can be difficult to relate this to stress, as these are all symptoms that are associated with ageing and that appear seemingly unrelated.

When signs gradually develop over a period of years it almost becomes the norm, and of course there is the oft-repeated phrase 'You're not getting any younger' – but age is not a medical diagnosis, nor need it be accepted as such.

Address the cause

Spend time and work out just exactly what the causes of your stress are. Although this seems obvious, it is probably the most effective way to reduce stress levels. If there is a particularly stressful situation, or a person (usually a work or family situation), address it head on. There is no need to be aggressive, but merely explain the circumstances to the person concerned, or, if it is a situation, change it. Focus on a time plan, because, as we have said, time is not a tangible entity and it can be used – to *your* advantage – as you consider appropriate. Time mismanagement is stressful in itself.

Say 'no'

'No' is probably the most difficult expression in the English language, and certainly the cause of much stress and distress. In fact, the word 'no' is rarely used in the Japanese language; although the word does exist it is considered rude to say 'no', so there are various ways of refusing without using the actual word. For example, 'This can be done' and 'I will come to that later' are ways of circumventing the problem in a polite manner. It is really saying, 'It can be done, but in my time and not necessarily now.' Other ways of addressing the problem are by suggesting a solution, or simply saying, 'I wish I could do that but . . .'

Talk, talk, talk

Talking is probably the most effective way of releasing your emotions, and pent-up emotions are a sure-fire guarantee that increased stress hormones and stress levels will follow. Unfortunately, men don't usually talk about feelings, unlike their female counterparts, and this is probably why men have much higher stress levels.

There is no Superman

There is no perfect man and it is certainly not you. Try to be the best you can but don't try to be something that you are not and cannot achieve. Everybody messes up, even the seemingly most perfect of humans, but trying to achieve the impossible is just another guaranteed way of increasing stress.

Exercise

Exercise is an essential way of relieving stress levels. Make the time and you will find it will repay you a hundredfold. You simply can't contemplate stressful emotions when you are exercising (unless you are Superman), so just do it.

Breathing

The importance of breathing in relaxation was fully discussed earlier in the book, and it is an essential technique in the management of stress. As we have already seen, the development of breathing exercises and techniques is of essential importance, as it is the only function that our body performs that is under both conscious and unconscious control. This fact, associated with the anatomical position of the respiratory centre in the brain next to that of the cardiac centre, means you can exert influence on your whole body simply by relaxing into a state of steady and even breathing at a rate of 6–8 breaths per minute. This obviously is very difficult, as we have seen. However, it can be achieved over time and is particularly promoted by meditation and relaxation techniques. In so doing, you not only control your breathing but you can control your heart rate and emotions – and therefore your stress levels.

Quiet time

Make a conscious effort to set aside five minutes of quiet time, at least once and preferably twice per day. Close your eyes and clear your mind of all conscious thought. Concentrate on nothing and listen to your breathing. After four or five minutes, slowly open your eyes and gradually – not suddenly – contemplate your surroundings.

Five minutes a day can make all the difference. Make the time.

Leave work at work

The mistake that most men make is to take work home with them, and, even worse, think about it all the time. While being diligent is to be commended, be realistic. Once again, focus your time on what can be done and then stop, and, most importantly, stop thinking about it. You don't get any medals for arriving at the morgue too early.

Create your own space

You need time and space for yourself. Even simply closing the door of the office at lunchtime for ten minutes and quietly meditating (not thinking about work) has been shown to have major effects on the improvement of many objective measures of health, such as heart rate and blood pressure. Remember, mental ill health can cause just as much *physical* damage to your body as physical ill health.

Relax

Relaxation is probably the most difficult attribute to achieve in life, because, although our bodies may relax, our minds never do. As we have already seen, it is important to chill out, make time for yourself and meditate. This means thinking about nothing. To help, you can use a heart-rate monitor, which gives a positive objective feedback, but merely practising focusing on your breathing has immense beneficial effects.

Drink up

Your body needs fluid – as water. One of the main secrets to health and the prevention of disease is making sure your body is fully hydrated at all times. This means drinking *before* you are thirsty. As we saw in Chapter 5, the body consists of about 72 per cent water, and we become thirsty after the loss of 1–3 per cent of body fluid. If this reaches 10 per cent, you die. So always have water available – probably the easiest way is to make sure that you have water constantly on your desk or near your working environment so that you physically see it and it reminds you to drink. The thirst mechanism is a very poor indicator of dehydration because it kicks in far too late. And, whenever the cells of the body are dehydrated, they are not functioning properly and are liable to become sick.

It is important not to fall into the trap of thinking that all fluids are the same. Fruit juices, beers and strong wines are high in sugar and therefore have an increased liability to produce the dreaded trio of diabetes, heart disease and hypertension. But, apart from these, alcohol in excess is very dangerous, as we saw in Chapter 6. It's not just cirrhosis of the liver, which everyone is aware of, but the widespread damage to the organs of the body caused by excess alcohol intake. And remember: excess can mean not just drinking too much at one time, but also the regularity of drinking alcohol on a daily basis.

Dehydration exacerbates many conditions:

- diabetes
- stress
- kidney disease
- hypertension
- headaches
- skin disorders

- constipation

- fatigue

- gall stones

- bowel disease

- palpitations

- arthritis

- mood swings

As an average, you should drink at least 500 ml of water every two hours, or 200 ml of water every 20 minutes during strenuous exercise. Alcohol, caffeine and refined carbohydrates all cause further loss of fluid – so you need to drink even more water when these are included in your diet.

Posture, posture, posture

Correct posture is essential for health. It forms the basis of your entire musculoskeletal system. Coordination, balance and muscle tone are all dependent on stable posture – in all bodily situations. Less commonly understood is that the function of the internal organs is also significantly dependent on posture, as the expansion of organs is an integral part of their healthy function. Breathing is an obvious example, but blood flow through the arteries and veins, movement of food through the bowel, and kidney function are similarly dependent on good posture.

The musculature of the body is based on the principle that for every agonist muscle there is an antagonist; in effect, this means that, if you have a muscle that performs one function across a joint, you need to have a muscle performing exactly the opposite on the other side of the joint to achieve muscular stability. We discussed posture and the two types of muscle in Chapter 8.

As we have already said, posture is part of everything you do. It is not just when you are sitting – although that is when most damage does tend to occur – but when you walk, exercise, and even lie in bed. Think 'posture' and you will address the problem, because the underlying issue is that we don't consider our posture. Most men in their forties or fifties develop some form of back pain, and this is almost always attributable to poor posture, which causes muscle strain and spasm insidiously – usually over a period of many years. However, there is a positive aspect: although there may be some permanent damage there is always a significant degree of pain due to a *developing* situation, which is still at a reversible stage, so the sooner you address the problem of poor posture, the better. Posture correction is cost-neutral and has only beneficial effects.

Quite simply, the human body is designed to be straight, not bent or hunched. It responds well to angles of 180 degrees or 90 degrees – and responds poorly to acute or obtuse angles. Simple strategies can produce amazing results.

- When upright – either standing or walking – always consciously pull your shoulders back and lift your head. Never stoop or hunch. This simple strategy draws the body naturally into the balanced position, with pressure and emphasis on the musculature distributed equally on each side of the body. It releases muscle imbalance in the back – especially the upper back – and allows more room for expansion of the internal organs.

- When seated at a desk, once again never stoop or hunch your shoulders – the classic position for upper-back and neck disorders, which are obviously exacerbated by prolonged computer use. Even with good posture, don't spend more than one hour constantly at a computer. Schedule other tasks to break the prolonged period before returning.

- If seated (not at a desk or computer), don't make the common mistakes of poor posture: legs crossed, legs straight but turned outwards, or – the commonest, yet again – stooping. Sit straight (but relaxed) with head up. It seems unnatural, but it is actually the most natural posture for the body and the muscles that support this position will develop strength the more it is adopted. Remember: the body musculature is designed for equal emphasis on both sides of the body. Curved or bent posture in early years will ensure a permanently bent posture later.

Muscle up

Remember, when we discuss muscle we are not talking only about the skeletal muscle that covers your body, but all of the muscular system:

- skeletal muscle

- smooth muscle

- cardiac muscle

When you exercise, either isotonically or isometrically, you increase the perfusion, i.e. supply, of blood to the muscles and, therefore, not only do you supply the muscles with the essential nutrients and oxygen that they need, but, much more importantly, you also remove the toxins and waste products. Of equal importance is that increasing blood flow removes the toxins from all of the organs of the body and therefore prevents the development of insidious diseases in organs that you would not have assumed initially were associated with exercise. So physical exercise not only improves skeletal muscle function (the muscles that you see) but also cardiac muscle function, because, obviously, it similarly improves blood flow to the heart muscle. You are not only exercising your skeletal muscles but also your cardiac muscles with moderate aerobic exercise.

And, of course, it is similarly important to exercise the smooth muscle in the gastrointestinal system of the body. This is partially affected by muscular exercise, because good posture and good blood flow will improve the health of the internal organs; but it is also particularly improved by diet. Eating a diet with high fibre content stretches the bowel and causes it to be much healthier. So you can see that exercising muscle involves much more than the usual 'muscle-up' exercises associated with cardio and weights. Diet is equally effective, not only in stretching the bowel and so stretching the smooth muscles, but also in providing the essential nutrients you need for healthy muscular function: skeletal, cardiac and smooth.

Exercising safely

But how should we exercise safely? This really depends on your state of fitness at the beginning of the programme. If you are completely unfit, then start slowly and build up gradually. The 'no pain, no gain' mantra is only for those who want an early heart attack. Start with a simple isometric exercise programme (see page 130) and perform this on at least four or five days per week. Couple this with either walking for twenty minutes per day, five days a week, or substitute swimming for one session of walking.

After one month, gradually introduce isotonic exercises (see page 141) but, most importantly, use low weights initially. Once again, it is very simple to make the mistake of assuming that, if you start with heavier weights, you will improve your fitness more rapidly. Nothing could be further from the truth. *Lower* weights with *more repetitions* are a far better way of increasing fitness initially. Then you can step up gradually to heavier weights as you progress – but at slow increments.

Those of you who are already engaged in exercise will have some knowledge of the best programme for you. What I would suggest is that, if you are engaging in isotonic exercises with mixed machines initially, or cardiovascular exercises, you really should include an isometric muscle programme, because isometric exercises complement isotonic exercises. The advantage of the isometric exercise is that it maintains the muscle at its resting length (see page 128), which of course is the length at which maximum power and fitness can be achieved. So, while isotonic exercises are undoubtedly important and have specific characteristics in themselves, the addition of isometric exercises does complement the isotonics.

But remember always to follow the simple stretching programme previously described (see page 142) before any exercise programme. This is particularly important if you are unaccustomed to exercise, as muscle strains and injuries can undoubtedly be caused by 'too much, too soon'.

Strenuous physical exercise is not essential, but can often be very enjoyable. What is essential is exercise of *some* form. Even walking three times a week for twenty minutes produces immense improvements in cardiovascular health and, generally unrecognised, immense benefits in reduction of stress and therefore the reduction of illness. Stretching is relatively simple, provided you don't *overstretch*, and can prevent muscle spasm, thereby delaying the development of arthritis and muscular pains, which are an inevitable feature of ageing at some time. The majority of muscle and joint problems are caused by spasm of the muscle; if you can reduce that spasm you will reduce the progression of the condition to a significant degree. Even if you are not too interested in exercise, make some time either to walk or swim on a regular basis. The health benefits are immense.

Putting the advice into practice

Let us summarise some of what we've learned so far. As discussed in the earlier chapters, the four essential areas that you need to address to achieve a real and sustainable health revolution are:

- food awareness, including a healthy approach to fluid balance

- heart protection
- stress relief
- muscular control

Now you need to position these complementary factors into the context of *your* lifestyle and *your* daily schedule. Everyone has different aspirations and different opinions of what is important for them, so only *you* can make the final decision. To do this we are going to use the 'Mars bar' mantra, because we have to look at work, rest and play. All of the above-mentioned factors (diet, heart protection, stress relief and muscular control) are an integral part of all you do in all situations, and you can choose to take control.

At work, the adrenal glands are under constant stress. Cortisol levels are high due to hectic lifestyles and constraints on time, and this leads to high blood pressure and all of the potential health hazards that can follow. As we saw in detail earlier, a fast pace of life often results in unhealthy food intake with resultant elevation of insulin levels, high blood pressure and increase risked of heart disease and diabetes.

At rest, the relaxed phase often involves an increase in alcohol intake, a lack of exercise and an increased intake of highly processed (unhealthy) foods such as crisps, chips and confectionary.

And 'men at play' can range from the sedentary act of TV gazing to active sports (e.g. tennis or cycling) or the gym. Social interactions often involve unhealthy activities:

- High consumption of alcohol.

- Unhealthy evening meals, either takeaway or ready meals, both high in processed foods, usually incorporating large amounts of trans fats.

- Of course, some men in this age range do participate in sports with an emphasis on cardiovascular exercise (such as cycling), but it is not the norm.

Reversing this inevitable progression towards ill health and poor quality of life requires lifestyle adjustment. The various strands for health have been described and can be simply addressed. The secret is to create your personalised daily time cycle.

As we have already discussed, there is no single, all-encompassing, perfect plan that will fit everyone. There are different levels of fitness, different tastes in diet and different approaches to our daily lives. However, it is certainly not only possible, but relatively straightforward, to formulate a series of principles on which an action plan can be based, and which have proven efficacy and success. The plan incorporates four main parts, all of which are complementary and all of which are essential:

- Establish a rationale for embarking on the programme.

- Create a food diary.

- Activate the plan.

- Evaluate the ongoing results.

Establish your personal rationale for health

This means you have to work out why you really want to become healthy and participate in this programme. It is not enough to have nebulous concepts such as 'I want to be healthy' or 'I want to live longer'. If this is the rationale, forget it now, because you will not be able to develop the motivation to continue, and it is important to realise – as I have emphasised constantly – that this is a lifestyle programme, not a quick fix. It is designed to make you healthy for the rest of your life, not just to lose weight or establish muscle in the short term. So, unless you can establish your aims and goals, and work out how you intend to achieve these, the rest is history. The main questions to ask are the following (and we would suggest that you photocopy this page, and physically write out the results on the dotted lines and retain them):

What is my main motivation to take action?

....

Before commencing the plan, are there any current health issues to be taken into consideration? If there are, discuss these with your medical practitioner before commencing.

....

Do you have any unhealthy lifestyle habits that you have embraced in the past?

....

Can you realistically deal with the restructuring of your daily lifestyle?

....

Can you set yourself a realistic goal by incorporating small changes on a regular basis?

....

Do you have someone to help you achieve this new action plan and change your lifestyle?

....

What are your expectations and are they realistic?

....

It is essential to realise that you need to be your own prime motivator in implementing any plan that is going to change your lifestyle, particularly one where your health is involved. Unless the main motivation comes from you, it won't work. Write your own answers honestly to these questions, and file for future reference, because we will be evaluating them later on.

Keep a diary: food, exercise and stress relief

Food planner

Using a daily food planner is essential to successful implementation of the action plan. In my experience with patients, food diaries have two main advantages.

- They are cathartic. In other words, they can help you realise exactly how your diet can be controlling your life.

- They enable you to identify the problem times in the day when inappropriate food choices are made, and therefore allow you to correct the problem areas.

In order to achieve this, you have to actually create a specific food diary in either a notebook or a template on the computer with several essential, itemised informational points, such as:

- Date.

- Time of day.

- Quantity of food. This is simply a generalised assessment of how much in weight, size or number you have eaten.

- Type of food. A simple description of the meal, breaking down the individual components. Always include sauces and gravy and also add 'extras' such as mayonnaise, salad dressing, sour cream or ketchup.

- Where you were at the time. Were you at home, for instance, or at the office, in a restaurant . . . ?

- What you were doing. For example, working, watching TV or travelling in the car.

- Whether you were alone or with someone – a partner, the family, friends.

- Mood. This information is essential, as mood can play a major part in eating habits.

A typical example of a food diary is as follows:

Date	Time	How much	Type of food	Where	Activity	Alone or with someone	Mood

There are a number of important points to remember in completing your food journal:

- **Do it now** Keep a record at the time, and don't depend on memory at the end of the day, as it is often at fault.

- **Include everything** Extras such as sauces, dressings, gravy can make a difference. Unless you follow the previous rules and write out everything you do as you go along, such items as crisps, sweets and chocolate can be missed and can soon add up.

- **Try to estimate the amount**. You don't need to be exact, but try to estimate what you are consuming, because it is much more helpful to have *some* idea of the amount.

- **Be honest**. You can help yourself only if you are honest with yourself. Small inaccuracies can have a major impact on health.

Undertaking a new lifestyle regime can be daunting, but recording all of your everyday experiences in detail can have immense advantages:

- accountability to yourself

- actually seeing your daily food intake, in detail, in black and white

- becoming aware of the types of food you are eating, and those that perhaps you *should* be including

- creating awareness of the nutritional values of the food that you are consuming

- the realisation of how much you are actually eating

- similarly, how much exercise you are committing yourself to and, more importantly, how much you are actually doing

- increasing your ability to make healthy choices by consciously reading the labels on bought foods

- awareness of food preparation, timescales and therefore the ability to schedule it into your programme

- becoming more organised, and particularly in relation to menu planning

- inevitably enjoying a higher standard of nutritionally based food

- allowing you the opportunity to make subtle changes to your daily food plan and enabling you to ease yourself into a healthy lifestyle

- identifying the 'dangerous hours'

- realisation of the amount of snacks and unnecessary food intake

- enjoying foods that you like to eat, but perhaps you did not realise how healthy they were

- making decisions on the daily plan that suits your lifestyle

- enabling you to schedule exercise programmes into your lifestyle by placing the same emphasis on exercise as you do on your professional life

- realisation that time for mental rest is as important as time for physical rest, and scheduling this into the daily programme

Exercise diary

Keep a record of dates, times and types of exercise on a daily basis. And record the following measurements before commencing and at two-week intervals thereafter:

- chest measurement

- waist measurement

- hip measurement

- upper-arm circumference

- upper-thigh circumference

It is amazing how motivating the objective perception of muscle improvement can be.

Stress relief

Keep a daily record of dates/times allocated to meditation and mental relaxation.

The daily action plan

Being proactive on a daily basis and creating small but subtle changes to your nutritional and exercise routine will improve your health in weeks, not years. I agree it is impossible to encompass everyone's daily lifestyle, diets and expectations, but I hope to show you how easy it is to implement small changes to your nutritional and exercise regime that not only make you healthier, but make you *feel* much healthier very quickly. All the principles have been described in previous chapters; this plan is really just to pull these together in a way that suits most people, or can be made to suit most people. However, you need to adapt it to your own specific needs. Of course, these are only suggestions; the options have been provided in detail (and with considerable variety) in Appendix A.

7 a.m. – starting the day

Exercise. The beginning of the day is an excellent time to incorporate an isometric exercise programme which involves no active stretching, can be embarked on immediately with no risk of injury, and increases muscle strength exponentially (page 130).

A healthy breakfast is an excellent start to the day, stabilising energy levels over a period of 4–6 hours and therefore removing the need to snack later in the morning.

Option 1: Scrambled eggs with smoked salmon

This is easily and quickly prepared, especially if you use a microwave, and provides energy for hours.

Carbohydrate content per serving: 0 grams

Option 2: Bacon and eggs

Obviously, this is more applicable when there is a little more time, such as at weekends, but is similarly nutritious and healthy.

Carbohydrate content per serving: 0 grams

11 a.m. – a dangerous hour

It's time to banish old routines and skip the snacks. If you have managed to establish your blood sugar at a stable level by having a breakfast as described above, then snacking will not be a temptation. If you must snack, then have a better breakfast the next day, but in the interim feast on nuts (such as hazelnuts, almonds or Brazils) or have some crudités with humus, both of which will stabilise blood sugar.

12.30–2 p.m. – time for lunch

Lunch is a time to re-energise (avoiding carbohydrates) and exercise the mind.

Option 1: Lunch at a restaurant

Fish and shellfish are always safest, as these stabilise the blood sugar and don't cause postprandial lethargy. Obviously, it is relatively simple to choose from the huge variety available in the recipes in Appendix A. Cod fillet with herb salad or stir-fried tiger prawns with chilli would be ideal candidates.

Carbohydrate content per serving: 0 grams

Option 2: Lunch on the run

Lunch on the run is nowhere near as difficult as you would imagine. Of course, we are presented with fast-food outlets selling foods that are all carbohydrate-based, such as burgers, pizzas, pasta or sandwiches, but there is a huge variety of options out there, many of which are incredibly healthy. It is not necessary to take your own lunch, as delis exist almost everywhere, with a wonderful selection of salads based on fish, such as tuna or salmon, or an unlimited variety of meats and salad options, all topped off with full-fat mayonnaise or dressings.

> Carbohydrate content per serving: 0–5 grams

1.30 p.m. – stress relief

The lunch period is a perfect time for stress relief. Adapt a 5–7-minute programme (see page 53) in a quiet part of the office or home, and this will have immense advantages to your concentration process for the rest of the afternoon.

3.30–4 p.m. – another danger period

Once again, if you are hypoglycaemic and snacking at this time of day, you simply haven't included the correct foods at lunch. In the interim, it is important to banish the old routine, cut out caffeine and replace with either tea or bottled water. Remember: dehydration is one of the most important contributors to inappropriate hunger. If you really do need snacks, once again nuts are the answer and not carbohydrates.

4.30–6.30 p.m. – yet another danger period

These are the really important times when you have finished work and are peckish and hypoglycaemic, and inevitably rush straight for something instantly gratifying, such as the old carb favourites: biscuits or crisps. To avoid the carb trap, have food prepared and ready that you can eat instantly. Potential options include:

■ smoked salmon with some lemon juice, prepared instantly, kills hunger instantly and will satisfy you for hours

■ cold chicken, preferably on the bone, once again satisfies hunger and stabilises blood sugar instantly

■ cheese with perhaps a little non-sweetened pickle, but with a maximum of two crackers

All of these will remove the overwhelming urge to consume carbohydrates, usually in inappropriate quantities.

6.30–7 p.m. – exercise

Exercise can be scheduled at any time between 6.30 and 9 p.m., depending on your normal daily work schedule, but *isotonic* exercises are particularly beneficial at this time of day. As you have stabilised your blood sugar with a non-carbohydrate source, such as smoked salmon or chicken, you will have enough energy to perform exercise – and not experience the intense hypoglycaemia afterwards. Of course, exercise can be performed either at home or at the gym, depending on your personal preferences, but it is important not to binge on carbohydrates immediately before exercise, as this can cause significant sugar imbalance. Before you start worrying about whether you will get enough energy from protein rather than carbohydrate, remember that rather lithe animal the cheetah, which manages to run at 70 miles an hour but has never eaten a carbohydrate in its life.

7–9 p.m. – dinner

Obviously the timing of dinner depends entirely on your personal lifestyle but it needs to be scheduled in as an important meal, which should be satisfying but not substantial. The options vary as to whether you eat out at a restaurant (see page 180) or at home, and typical options would be:

- Chargrilled Tuna Steaks with Oriental Dressing
  (page 254) – *carbohydrate content per serving: 7 grams*

- Moroccan Lamb
  (page 265) – *carbohydrate content per serving: 1 gram*

- Oven-baked Ricotta with Vine-ripened Cherry Tomatoes
  (page 284) – *carbohydrate content per serving: 4 grams*

And, of course, never forget the ubiquitous omelettes, such as:

- Green Apple and Roquefort Omelette
  (page 275) – *carbohydrate content per serving: 5 grams*

- Mushroom Omelette
  (page 274) – *carbohydrate content per serving: 5 grams*

9–10 p.m. – stress relief

The end of the day is an essential time for stress relief in order to reduce mental overactivity before sleep. Meditation is an excellent natural sedative.

Evaluate, evaluate, evaluate

Evaluation is the key to success, and it is important to schedule in regular evaluation steps at fortnightly intervals to avoid complacency – which always leads to failure. To prevent plateaux – or reverses – you need to evaluate each individual component of the four-stage process:

Motivation for embarking on the programme

Complete the evaluation form you initially completed before embarking on the programme (page 214) and compare each of the individual points before and after. It is essential to re-evaluate each of the individual parameters to determine whether your goals are really being achieved and, if not, how to achieve them.

Diet

Evaluate your diet (via the food diary) on a daily basis, and in particular compare your ability to maintain the programme at the commencement of the programme with two weeks later. Assess the weight change after the initial two-week evaluation period.

Exercise

Once again, examine the daily diary to determine whether the exercise programme has been achieved. Compare the essential measurements of chest, waist, thigh and upper arm and calculate the percentage changes before and after.

Subjectively assess your increase in energy after the programme in comparison with before, as a percentage.

Stress relief

Once again, examine the daily programme to determine whether you have managed to comply with the two periods of stress-relief meditation per day as suggested and, if not, why not. Subjectively assess whether your stress patterns are improved and you have improved concentration.

This is, of course, only the beginning. It is important to realise that, during the initial two weeks, you have to reverse some of the unfortunate trends that have developed over many years before you can begin to see positive results. Further improvement will undoubtedly occur in future two-week cycles, so it is important not to become complacent after the first two weeks, but rather to reinforce the initial success with a continued daily diary of diet, exercise and stress relief and to assess this at two-weekly intervals to determine progress. You will undoubtedly be successful in the initial fortnight of the programme, but it is important to realise that complacency is the ultimate killer for health.

You don't have to be perfect but you *do* need to be conscientious. As you can see, we have inserted into the time slots a series of suggested meals and exercise programmes for both the mind and the body that are eminently applicable to most lifestyles, but the important part is that:

- this is only a suggested cycle

- it doesn't apply to everyone and won't necessarily apply to you

Use this template of the cycle and insert into the various time slots the areas that are particularly applicable to you: the foods, the exercise regime and the mental exercises that you can fit into your own daily programme on a regular basis.

It is essential to emphasise that this is a *cycle*, not a *list*. A cycle is ongoing, and never stops. However, a list has to be commenced afresh for each individual day. This is an ongoing cycle and not a stop/start progression that will inevitably come to an end. The cycle becomes just that: as you programme your body to reduce its addiction to carbohydrates, and therefore reduce the risk of heart disease, diabetes and hypertension, the wheel keeps on turning in a self-sustaining manner without any willpower or input from you. The secret is to start with an empty timetable and complete the slots on the wheel with a schedule *appropriate to you and individualised for you.* You can then start the wheel turning, because once it is revolving it should become a perpetual motion. You have simply removed the restrictions of poor diet and lifestyle on your quality of life.

SUMMARY

▶ Remember that you are what you eat, so cut out processed foods and the bread, pasta and rice. They're not good for you. Replace them with vegetables and salad.

▶ Look after your heart through diet, reducing your stress levels and doing exercise.

▶ Men are much more likely to be unaware of their stress levels than women. Unexplained headaches, onset of indigestion, reduced sex drive and depression are all early signs. So learn to recognise these signs of stress.

▶ Make sure you keep hydrated. Don't wait for the thirst signal. Pre-empt it. Drink 500 ml of water every two hours.

▶ Even walking three times a week for twenty minutes produces immense improvements in cardiovascular health.

▶ Correct posture is essential for health. It forms the basis of your entire musculoskeletal system.

▶ Strenuous physical exercise isn't essential, but you must do exercise in *some* form.

▶ Create your personalised Daily Time Cycle.

Recipes for Life

Vegetables are very nutritious, containing many essential vitamins and minerals that are not present in foods of animal origin. They supply essential vitamins, such as A, C, E and K, which are either absent or present in such low quantities in foods of animal origin that it is virtually impossible to obtain them except from vegetables.

However, it is important to realise that the converse is also true. For example, with the exception of soya products (such as tofu), no other vegetable product contains all of the essential amino acids that we require for health. In addition to a deficiency in essential amino acids (the building blocks of proteins), other essential nutrients in our diet, such as iron, are present only in small quantities in the vegetable kingdom. In order to obtain the same amount of iron from broccoli as you would obtain from meat, you would need to consume 2 kg of broccoli to 100 grams of meat products.

In other words, the amount you restrict meats or animal-based products from your diet will determine how many supplements you require.

A balance between vegetables and foods of some animal origin (which could be eggs or fish) is by far the healthiest combination. If you don't eat meat at all in any form, then combining grains with dairy products is the safest option. The following recipes have been deliberately chosen to provide as wide a range of vitamins as possible, but obviously it is impossible to provide a comprehensive vegetarian option in a book of this size. Provided you have the general principles (described above), you can easily remain perfectly healthy and fit on a vegetarian diet; however, adding some non-meat products (such as fish or eggs) does provide the essential amino acids otherwise lacking in a vegetarian programme. It is important to realise that vitamin B_{12} does not exist anywhere in the plant kingdom and therefore if you are entirely vegan then you must take vitamin B_{12} supplements.

WAKE-UP STARTERS

Juices and smoothies are excellent sources of nutrition but unfortunately tend to have higher carb content due to the fructose in fruit. And they are often not sufficiently satisfying to stave off hunger until lunch. So if you find juices and smoothies sufficient for breakfast that's fine, but if you need something more substantial you can combine the starter *with* a breakfast – provided you select one that is low in carbs to offset the higher-carb smoothie. For example, citrus compote with scrambled eggs would be 19 grams of carbs, but citrus compote with porridge would equal a disastrous 37 grams – not the perfect start to the day.

Citrus Compote

SERVES 2

1 lime
1 blood orange
1 medium grapefruit
200g natural yoghurt
1 tbsp fresh mint leaves, chopped

- Grate the rind of the lime and orange and set aside.
- Peel the lime and orange and grapefruit, and segment the fruits.
- Mix together the citrus fruits with the yoghurt, and garnish with mint leaves and rind.

Carbohydrate content per serving: 17 grams

Orange-and-Ginger Reviver

SERVES 2

2 tbsp fresh ginger, grated
2 fresh oranges, peeled and chopped

- Combine the orange with the ginger, blend and serve immediately.

Carbohydrate content per serving: 13 grams

Beetroot Booster

SERVES 2

2 celery stalks, chopped
4 baby beetroots, peeled and sliced
100g watercress, trimmed
200ml water

- Blend the celery, beetroot and watercress.
- Stir in the water and serve.

Carbohydrate content per serving: 7 grams

Classic Berry Surprise

SERVES 2

6 large strawberries
3 tbsp blueberries
3 tbsp raspberries
150ml water
sprig of fresh mint

- Blend the berries.
- Stir in the cold water.
- Serve, garnished with a sprig of mint.

Carbohydrate content per serving: 7 grams

Mint and Watermelon Refresher

SERVES 2

900g watermelon peeled
10 fresh mint leaves

- Blend the watermelon with the mint and serve.

Carbohydrate content per serving: 22 grams

Carrot and Orange Juice

SERVES 2

1 large orange, peeled and segmented
1 large carrot, peeled and chopped
100ml water
4 ice cubes (optional)

- Blend the orange and carrot, stir in the water and ice, and serve.

Carbohydrate content per serving: 15 grams

Immune-boosting Juice

SERVES 2

5 kiwi fruit, peeled and sliced
150g green grapes, seedless
100ml water

• Blend the kiwi fruit with the grapes, stir in the water and serve.

Carbohydrate content per serving: 23 grams

Spicy Smoothie

SERVES 2

200ml carrot juice
3 large plum tomatoes, skin removed, deseeded and chopped
1tbsp freshly squeezed lime juice
1 celery stick, sliced
50g baby spinach leaves, stalks removed
1 tbsp fresh flat-leaf parsley leaves, chopped
1 tsp curry powder
4 ice cubes
100ml spring water

• Blend the ingredients and serve immediately.

Carbohydrate content per serving: 12 grams

BREAKFAST

Breakfast is an essential part of the day, and you need to incorporate this into your schedule as a priority if you are going to be successful. Of course, some individuals don't need – or don't like – breakfast, and that's fine, provided they plan to eat at a suitable time later and don't allow hunger to develop, because the basis of the programme is the avoidance of hypoglycaemia. For the rest of us, breakfast is essential to stabilise our metabolism and hormonal balance for the day ahead.

As we have seen, it doesn't require much time to have a quick, nutritious and stabilising breakfast, but it does require a little planning and forethought – and commitment. You may be surprised to see there are some recipes that include toast for breakfast (absolute maximum of one small slice); this is to allow those who simply can't exist without bread an option. There is even a breakfast tortilla. But there are far more healthy potential options from the immense list of nutritious foods included without restriction, so keep to the healthy choices as much as possible. It's far better to avoid the higher-GI meals if possible, and definitely for the first two weeks, but a slice of toast at breakfast will not ruin the programme provided you are careful to adhere strictly to low-GI foods for the rest of the day.

Porridge with Blueberries

SERVES 2

450ml water, boiled
4 tbsp oatmeal
1 tsp sugar (optional)
8 tbsp full-cream milk
2 tbsp blueberries

- Pour the water into a medium saucepan and bring to the boil, then stir in the oatmeal.
- Simmer gently for 20 minutes.
- Stir in the sugar (if desired) and milk, add the blueberries and serve.

Carbohydrate content per serving: 20 grams

Scrambled Eggs

SERVES 2

4 large free-range eggs
2 tbsp full-cream milk
30g butter
pinch of sea salt
freshly ground black pepper

- Beat the eggs with milk in a medium mixing bowl and season to taste.
- Melt the butter in a medium saucepan over a low heat and add the eggs. Stir constantly for about 2–3 minutes.

- Remove from the heat before the eggs have set, and serve immediately.

Scrambled eggs can be cooked quickly in the morning by a microwave technique, as follows.

- Beat the eggs as described, then pour into a microwave-safe bowl and place in the centre of the microwave oven. Set the oven to high and cook for about 1 minute.
- Stir the mixture and then repeat this process twice and serve immediately.

As with omelettes, the options for adding delicious accompaniments to scrambled eggs is almost limitless:

30g grated Emmental or Jarlsberg cheese

40g smoked salmon, sliced finely

1 large plum tomato, seeded and diced

Parma ham, finely sliced

1 tbsp fresh basil leaves, chopped finely

Carbohydrate content per serving: 2 grams

Poached Eggs

....

SERVES 2

4 large free-range eggs

- Add boiling water to a shallow saucepan, and then reduce the heat to simmer.
- Slide each egg individually into the water.
- Allow to poach for about 3 minutes, and then remove the eggs from the water with a perforated spoon.
- Serve immediately on a slice of buttered wholegrain toast (optional).

Once again, the microwave option is less time-consuming.

- Break each egg into the plastic containers specifically designed for microwave egg poaching.
- Pierce the top if the yolks 3–4 times with a sharp knife, spoon over a teaspoon of cold water and close the sealed top of the container.
- Cook on medium (never high) for 1–2 minutes and allow to stand for 1 minute before serving.

> Carbohydrate content per serving: nil (17 g with toast)

Mushrooms on Toast

SERVES 2

150g button mushrooms
50g unsalted butter
1 tbsp chopped fresh basil leaves
1 tbsp chopped fresh oregano leaves
pinch of rock salt
freshly ground black pepper
1 slice wholegrain toast (optional)

- Wipe the mushrooms, then halve them lengthwise.
- Heat the butter in a medium saucepan and sauté the mushrooms for about 2–3 minutes.
- Stir in the herbs and seasoning and heat through for another further minute before serving on a slice of wholegrain toast (optional).

Carbohydrate content per serving: 18 grams
(1 g without toast)

Wholemeal Cheese Toasty

SERVES 2

2 slices wholegrain bread
50g grated cheese (of choice, however Emmental, Jarlsberg and
    Edam are excellent)
pinch of rock salt
freshly ground black pepper

- Lightly toast the wholegrain bread.
- Top with grated cheese and cook under the grill until the cheese
    has melted.
- Season to taste and serve immediately.

Of course, once again, the toasted-cheese potential accompaniments are restricted only by your imagination:

plum tomato, seeded and diced

spring onion, chopped finely

1 tsp Worcester sauce

half a small green chilli, seeded and diced

prosciutto ham, diced

50g smoked salmon with 1tsp fresh dill leaves, chopped

Carbohydrate content per serving: 17–20 grams

Big Breakfast Tortilla

SERVES 2

4 large free-range eggs
2 tbsp full-cream milk
pinch of rock salt
freshly ground black pepper
30g unsalted butter
1 tbsp fresh flat-leaf parsley, chopped
1 tbsp fresh basil leaves, chopped
3 slices prosciutto ham, chopped
2 medium tortillas
25–30g watercress
1 plum tomato, diced

- Scramble the eggs (see page 234).

- Stir in the parsley, basil and prosciutto and season to taste.

- Wrap the tortillas in aluminium foil and heat in a hot oven for about 30–45 seconds.

- Place the watercress and tomato on each tortilla, topped with the scrambled-egg-and-prosciutto mixture and season to taste.

- Serve immediately.

Carbohydrate content per serving: 23 grams

Ham and Cheese Bagel

SERVES 2

1 medium bagel, halved
6 slices of Parma ham
50g Jarlsberg cheese, grated
1 tbsp fresh basil leaves, chopped
pinch of rock salt
freshly ground black pepper

- Heat the bagel halves in the oven for about 1 minute.
- Top each half with slices of Parma ham and Jarlsberg cheese.
- Grill until the cheese is melted, sprinkle over the basil, season to taste and serve.

Carbohydrate content per serving: 15 grams

Flat Mushrooms with Scrambled Eggs

SERVES 2

1 tbsp unsalted butter
1 tbsp wholegrain mustard
2 large flat mushrooms
4 large free-range eggs
1 tbsp freshly chopped flat-leaf parsley
pinch of rock salt
freshly ground black pepper

- Melt the butter in a medium saucepan and stir in the wholegrain mustard.

- Spread the mixture over the flat mushrooms and grill for about 2–3 minutes.

At the same time:

- Prepare the scrambled eggs (see page 234).

- Top the mushrooms with scrambled eggs and flat-leaf parsley, and season to taste.

Carbohydrate content per serving: 4 grams

POULTRY

Poultry does not restrict you to boring, pre-cooked chicken – useful though this is for a quick and nutritious snack. On the contrary, poultry can provide the basis for many diverse flavours, from game to turkey, duck to quail. And these are very simple to prepare, once again based on prior planning to ensure the necessary ingredients are available.

Oven-baked Duck with Tarragon Dressing

SERVES 2

2 medium duck breasts
100g mangetout

Tarragon dressing:

1 tsp wholegrain mustard
1 tbsp chopped fresh tarragon
1 tbsp extra-virgin olive oil
20ml red wine vinegar
1 tsp crushed black peppercorns
1 spring onion, chopped finely

- Place the duck breasts on a baking tray and cook in the centre of a preheated oven at 200°C (gas mark 5) for about 20 minutes.

- At the same time, lightly steam the mangetout for 5–7 minutes.

- Put the ingredients for the dressing into a small bowl and mix together.

- Serve the duck with mangetout and drizzle over the tarragon dressing.

Carbohydrate content per serving: 3 grams

Poached Chicken with Robust Red Wine

SERVES 2

2 tbsp extra-virgin olive oil
2 shallots, peeled and sliced
2 medium chicken breasts, approx. 150g each
2 small red peppers, deseeded and sliced finely
1 garlic clove, peeled and finely chopped
250g plum tomatoes, chopped
250ml robust red wine
1 tbsp fresh marjoram leaves
1 bay leaf

- Heat the olive oil in a large frying pan and sauté the shallots for about 2–3 minutes.

- Add the chicken and cook until browned.

- Add the peppers, garlic, tomatoes, wine, marjoram and bay leaf to the pan. Cover and simmer for about 45 minutes.

- Serve immediately with salad (see page 277).

Carbohydrate content per serving: 11 grams

Chargrilled Chicken with Chilli Salsa

SERVES 2

2 chicken breasts (approximately 150g each)
3 tbsp extra-virgin olive oil
4 tbsp freshly squeezed lemon juice
1 tsp lemon rind
pinch of sea salt
freshly ground black pepper

Salsa:

12 cherry tomatoes, finely chopped
1 small red chilli, deseeded and chopped finely
1 garlic clove, peeled and chopped finely
2 tbsp extra-virgin olive oil
1 tbsp freshly squeezed lime juice
pinch of sea salt
freshly ground black pepper

- Mix together the extra-virgin olive oil with the lemon juice and lemon rind, season to taste and brush over the chicken.

- Cook the chicken on a griddle pan for 6–8 minutes, turning once.

- At the same time mix together the ingredients of the salsa in a medium mixing bowl.

- Serve the chicken on a bed of wild rocket, topped with salsa and season to taste.

Carbohydrate content per serving: 8 grams

Spicy Grilled Chicken with Watercress

SERVES 2

2 medium chicken breast fillets (approximately 150g each)

Marinade:

100ml mirin (or dry sherry)
dash of Tabasco sauce (optional)
2cm fresh root ginger, peeled and grated
¼ tsp ground cumin
¼ tsp ground coriander
1 tbsp fresh basil leaves, chopped
2 shallots, peeled and finely diced
50ml chicken stock

100g watercress leaves
freshly ground black pepper
pinch of sea salt

- Mix together the ingredients of the marinade in a medium mixing bowl and marinade the chicken for at least one hour.
- Grill the chicken under a moderate heat for about 8 minutes per side, turning once.
- Serve the chicken on a bed of watercress, and season to taste.

Carbohydrate content per serving: 6 grams

Simple Chilli Turkey

SERVES 2

2 tbsp extra-virgin olive oil
2 medium turkey breasts, approx. 150g each, skin removed
1 medium red onion, peeled and chopped
4 medium tomatoes, diced
150ml vegetable stock
2 celery sticks, chopped into 2cm lengths
1 medium red pepper, deseeded and sliced
1 courgette, chopped on the diagonal
1 medium yellow squash, sliced finely
1 tsp hot chilli powder

- Heat the extra-virgin olive oil in a medium saucepan and sauté the turkey and onion for about 5 minutes.

- Stir in the tomatoes, stock, celery, pepper, courgette and squash with the chilli powder.

- Simmer gently for about 30 minutes and serve immediately.

Carbohydrate content per serving: 10 grams

Grilled Chicken with Harissa

SERVES 2

2 medium chicken breasts, approximately 150g each
1 tbsp harissa
1 tbsp freshly squeezed lemon juice

- Mix together the chicken breasts with the harissa and lemon juice in a medium mixing bowl, then grill for about 8 minutes, turning once.
- Set aside to cool, then slice thickly.
- Serve with Healthy Green Salad (see page 279).

Carbohydrate content per serving: 3 grams

FISH AND SHELLFISH

Fish and shellfish are simply the perfect foods in every possible way: delicious varied flavours; totally nutritious with essential amino acids, essential fatty acids, vitamins and minerals; and remarkably simple to prepare in tasty recipes, which can be on the table in minutes. For example, moules marinière (mussels) in white-wine bouillon takes five minutes to prepare and five minutes to cook – and tastes absolutely delicious. Or smoked salmon crêpes. Or stir-fried prawns with chilli mixed peppers. The sea provides the most delicious natural foods. Just add some simple natural flavours from herbs and seasoning for the perfect meal.

Citrus Scallops

SERVES 2

8 scallops
1 tbsp extra-virgin olive oil
1 blood orange, peeled and chopped
1 lemon, peeled and chopped
1 lime, peeled and chopped
1 tbsp fresh chives, snipped
1 tbsp fresh flat-leaf parsley leaves

Dressing:

1 tbsp orange juice
1 tbsp lime juice
1 tsp lemon rind
1 tbsp extra-virgin olive oil

- Heat 1 tbsp of extra-virgin olive oil in a medium frying pan, add the scallops and sauté gently for about 3 minutes, turning once, then set aside.

- Whisk together the ingredients of the dressing in a small bowl.
- Add the orange, lemon, lime and herbs to a salad bowl, toss with freshly squeezed lemon juice and black pepper.
- Drizzle over the dressing and toss gently.
- Serve the scallops on a bed of herb salad.

Carbohydrate content per serving: 5 grams

Crunchy Cod Fillets with Herb Salad

SERVES 2

2 medium cod fillets, approximately 150g each
1 tbsp extra-virgin olive oil

Basil-and-coriander salad

1 tbsp fresh basil leaves
1 tbsp fresh coriander leaves
1 tbsp fresh dill
100g wild rocket leaves
2 tbsp freshly squeezed lemon juice
freshly ground black pepper

- Place the cod in a baking dish, drizzle over the oil and bake in the centre of a preheated oven at 180°C (gas mark 4) for 20 minutes.
- Add together the contents of the basil-and-coriander salad in a large mixing bowl, drizzle over the lemon juice and toss gently.
- Serve the cod on a bed of basil-and-coriander salad, and season to taste.

Carbohydrate content per serving: 2 grams

Stir-fried Tiger Prawns with Chilli Mixed Peppers

SERVES 2

2 tbsp extra-virgin olive oil
1 garlic clove, peeled and chopped
2 spring onions, chopped
1 small red pepper, deseeded and sliced finely
1 small yellow pepper, deseeded and sliced finely
1 small red chilli, deseeded and chopped
250g cooked tiger prawns, peeled and de-veined
1 tbsp sweet sherry (or mirin)
pinch of sea salt
freshly ground black pepper
few drops of sesame oil
1 tbsp chopped fresh dill

- Heat the extra-virgin olive oil in a medium frying pan and sauté the garlic, spring onions, peppers and chilli for about 2 minutes.

- Stir in the cooked tiger prawns and sherry (or mirin).

- Season to taste and stir-fry for another minute.

- Then serve, drizzling over a splash of sesame oil and a handful of chopped dill.

Carbohydrate content per serving: 7 grams

Cooked Tiger Prawns with Seasonal Mixed Fruit

SERVES 2

10 cooked tiger prawns
½ small mango, peeled and sliced
2 kiwi fruit, peeled and sliced
1 tbsp orange juice

Dressing:

2 tbsp fresh mint leaves
1 tbsp fresh coriander leaves
1 garlic clove, peeled and chopped
2cm fresh ginger root, peeled and chopped
2 tbsp freshly squeezed lime juice
1 tbsp extra-virgin olive oil

- Toss the prawns with the mango, kiwi fruit and orange juice.
- Blend together the mint and coriander leaves with the garlic, ginger, lime juice and oil.
- Toss the prawn fruit salad in the dressing and serve immediately.

Carbohydrate content per serving: 20 grams

Smoked Salmon Sashimi

SERVES 2

100g smoked salmon, sliced finely
1 tsp wasabi sauce
½ Hass avocado, stone removed, peeled and sliced finely lengthwise
½ Lebanese cucumber, deseeded and sliced finely lengthwise
2 spring onions, sliced finely
¼ sheet of eaki-nori (seaweed), sliced into 1cm-wide strips
1 tsp sesame seeds, toasted
1 tbsp mirin
1 tbsp Japanese soy sauce

- Place half the salmon slices on a serving dish separately, add a little wasabi, then top each piece with slices of avocado, cucumber, and spring onion.

- Add a further salmon slice to make a 'salmon sandwich'.

- Wrap a single seaweed strip around each salmon sandwich.

- Sprinkle with toasted sesame seeds and drizzle over a little mirin.

- Serve with a separate bowl of soy sauce.

Carbohydrate content per serving: 1 gram

Fresh Mussel Salad with Aromatic Ginger Dressing

SERVES 2

750g fresh mussels, bearded and scrubbed
100g asparagus, trimmed
1 medium yellow pepper, deseeded and sliced finely
100g baby spinach leaves
2 tbsp fresh chives, snipped

Ginger dressing:

5cm fresh ginger root, peeled and grated
1 tbsp freshly squeezed lime juice
1 tbsp extra-virgin olive oil

- Wash and scrub the mussels, discarding any that are open or broken and don't close when tapped.
- Place the mussels in large saucepan, add water to almost cover the mussels and bring to the boil.
- Cover and lower the heat to simmer until the mussels open (usually 6–7 minutes).
- Remove the open mussels with a perforated spoon, and set aside.
- Steam the asparagus for about 5 minutes until tender.
- Mix together the fresh ginger, lime juice, and olive oil.
- Mix together the yellow pepper, spinach, fresh chives and mussels in a moderate mixing bowl.
- Serve immediately, having drizzled over the ginger dressing.
- Season to taste.

Carbohydrate content per serving: 3 grams

Chargrilled Tuna Steaks with Oriental Dressing

SERVES 2

2 medium tuna steaks, approximately 150g each
100g wild rocket leaves
1 small red pepper, sliced finely
1 small yellow pepper, sliced finely

Dressing:

1 green chilli, deseeded and finely chopped
1 spring onion, sliced finely
1 garlic clove, peeled and crushed
1 tbsp soy sauce
1 tsp mirin

- Grill the tuna on high heat for about 2 minutes on each side, then set aside.
- Whisk together the chilli, spring onion, garlic, soy sauce and mirin in a small bowl.
- Serve the tuna on a bed of rocket and peppers, and drizzle over the dressing.

Carbohydrate content per serving: 7 grams

White Sole Fillets with Herb Dressing

SERVES 2

100g broccoli florets
2 medium courgettes, sliced lengthways
1 tbsp extra-virgin olive oil
2 medium sole fillets
4 cherry tomatoes, chopped
1 tbsp lemon juice
1 tbsp fresh dill, chopped
1 tbsp fresh chives, snipped
Herb Dressing (see page 300)

- Steam the broccoli florets and courgettes for about 5 minutes until tender, then set aside.
- Heat the olive oil in a small frying pan and cook the sole for about 4 minutes, turning once.
- Remove from the pan and set aside.
- Add the tomatoes, lemon juice, dill and chives to the pan and cook for about 1 minute.
- Serve the sole with the tomatoes, broccoli and courgettes, drizzling the herb dressing over the fish.
- Season to taste.

Carbohydrate content per serving: 5 grams

Chargrilled Salmon with Asparagus

SERVES 2

2 tsp runny honey
1 tbsp light soy sauce
1 tsp wholegrain mustard
2 medium salmon fillets
2 tbsp extra-virgin olive oil
100g asparagus
30g Parmesan cheese, freshly grated
pinch of rock salt
freshly ground black pepper

- Mix together the honey, soy sauce and wholegrain mustard in a small bowl and coat the salmon fillets with the mixture.

- Heat the olive oil in a grill pan and chargrill the salmon fillets for about 4 minutes per side, turning once.

- At the same time, lightly steam the asparagus for about 4–5 minutes.

- Serve the salmon on the asparagus and top with Parmesan cheese.

- Season to taste.

Carbohydrate content per serving: 6 grams

Moules Marinière

....

SERVES 2

750g fresh mussels, bearded and scrubbed
1 tbsp fresh thyme, finely chopped
2 shallots, peeled and diced
150ml dry white wine
75g butter
freshly ground black pepper

- Wash and scrub the mussels, discarding any that are closed and do not open when tapped.
- Place the mussels in a large saucepan with the thyme, shallots and wine and bring to the boil.
- Cover and simmer for 5–6 minutes.
- Transfer the mussels to a shallow casserole and keep warm.
- Strain the remaining mixture, return to the pan and reduce by about half.
- Add the butter and simmer for 1–2 minutes, then pour over the mussels and serve immediately, seasoning to taste.

Carbohydrate content per serving: 2 grams

Crêpes

Crêpes alone don't come under the heading of fish and shellfish, of course, but bear with me. First we'll deal with making the crêpes, then we'll move on to more tasty dishes using crêpes with fish and shellfish.

These savoury crêpes can be made, either by purchasing the readymade variety, or by making your own. Making your own is incredibly simple and they taste delicious. Each crêpe contains only about 5–6 grams of carbohydrate (the equivalent of about a third of a slice of bread) and it is perfectly simple to include these in your low-GI programme.

Crêpes have the advantage of being perfect at any time of day, whether for breakfast, lunch or dinner. With a selection of fillings, they can be folded into triangles, or folded in half over the filling, or rolled around the filling.

Rather than explain the traditional method of making crêpes using a frying pan, which is a little more time-consuming, we suggest using a crêpe maker, which is very quick and simple.

250g plain flour, seasoned with a pinch of sea salt
1 large free-range egg, beaten
150ml full-cream milk
1 tbsp melted butter

- Sieve the seasoned flour into a medium mixing bowl.
- Whisk half of the beaten egg mixture into the flour.
- Gradually blend in the milk and the remaining egg, drawing the mixture to the centre of the bowl as you do so to achieve an even consistency.
- Allow to stand for 30–45 minutes.
- As you are about to cook, stir the melted butter into the mixture.

- Pour the mixture into a wide shallow dish.
- When the crêpe maker is hot, dip it horizontally into the mixture to coat lightly. As the edge of the crêpe becomes lightly brown, remove with a palette-knife and repeat for the next crêpe.

Smoked Salmon Crêpe

SERVES 2

100g smoked salmon, sliced finely
100g natural yoghurt
1 tbsp fresh chives, snipped
2 tbsp freshly squeezed lemon juice

- Make the crêpes as described in the previous recipe.
- Mix together the smoked salmon, yoghurt and chives in a medium mixing bowl.
- Place the salmon and yoghurt mixture on the crêpe and drizzle over lemon juice.
- Roll up the crêpe and serve.

Carbohydrate content per serving (per crêpe): 8 grams

Prawn and Mayonnaise Crêpes

SERVES 2

6 crêpes
120g peeled, cooked prawns
1 tbsp organic mayonnaise
2 tsp chopped fresh basil
2 tsp chopped fresh dill
freshly ground black pepper

- Prepare the crêpes as described on page 258.
- Mix together the prawns, mayonnaise, basil and dill in a medium mixing bowl and season to taste.
- Spoon the mixture over the crêpes, fold in half and serve.

Carbohydrate content per serving (per crêpe): 5 grams

Hearty Smoked Haddock Chowder

SERVES 2

1 tbsp butter
1 small potato, peeled and diced
1 fennel bulb, sliced finely
1 tbsp plain flour
200ml full cream milk
1 large smoked haddock fillet (approximately 150g), sliced
1 tbsp fresh dill, chopped
1 tbsp crème fraîche
1 tbsp freshly squeezed lemon juice
pinch of rock salt
freshly ground black pepper

- Melt the butter in a medium saucepan, and cook the potatoes and fennel over a low heat for 3–4 minutes.

- Stir in the flour.

- Stir in the milk slowly, then return to the boil, while stirring continuously.

- Simmer for 3–4 minutes and then add the sliced haddock and cook over a low heat for another 3–4 minutes.

- Stir in the dill, crème fraîche, lemon juice and seasoning.

- Heat through then serve immediately.

Carbohydrate content per serving: 17 grams

Whiting Fillets with Dry White Wine

SERVES 2

4 medium whiting fillets
1 tbsp butter
1 tbsp fresh dill, chopped
120ml dry white wine
pinch of sea salt
freshly ground black pepper

- Place the whiting in an ovenproof dish and top with butter cubes and the chopped dill.

- Pour the wine around the fish fillets, cover with pierced aluminium foil and cook in the centre of a preheated oven at 180°C (gas mark 4) for about 20 minutes.

- Season to taste and serve with Healthy Green Salad (see page 279).

Carbohydrate content per serving: 2 grams

Haddock with Coriander

....

SERVES 2

2 medium haddock fillets, approximately 150g each
1 tbsp crème fraîche
1 garlic clove, peeled and crushed
1 medium plum tomato, sliced
1 shallot, peeled and finely sliced
1 tbsp fresh coriander leaves, chopped
1 small red chilli, deseeded and diced finely
pinch of sea salt
freshly ground black pepper

- Place each fish fillet on aluminium foil in an ovenproof dish.

- Spread the crème fraîche and garlic over the fillets.

- Top with sliced tomato, shallots, coriander and chilli and season to taste.

- Close the foil parcels and bake in the centre of a preheated oven at 180°C (gas mark 4) for about 20 minutes.

- Serve with Healthy Green Salad (see page 279).

Carbohydrate content per serving: 5 grams

Grilled Tuna Steaks

....

SERVES 2

1 tbsp green peppercorns, crushed
3 tbsp freshly squeezed lime juice
2 tbsp extra-virgin olive oil
pinch of sea salt
2 medium tuna steaks, about 15g each
1 large free-range egg
1 garlic clove, peeled and chopped
125ml extra-virgin olive oil
2 tbsp fresh marjoram or oregano leaves, finely chopped

- Mix together the lime juice, 2 tbsp extra-virgin olive oil and pinch of sea salt with the peppercorns.

- Place the tuna steaks in a shallow dish and drizzle over the lime-and-olive-oil mixture.

- Set aside in the fridge overnight.

- Blend together the egg and garlic, and gradually pour the oil in slowly to create a mayonnaise. Blend until the mayonnaise has thickened.

- Grill the tuna for about 6 minutes, turning once.

- Serve immediately, garnished with the fresh herb leaves and spoon over the garlic mayonnaise.

- Serve with Healthy Green Salad (see page 279).

Carbohydrate content per serving: 3 grams

Poached Haddock with Dill and Chives

SERVES 2

2 smoked haddock fillets, approximately 150g each
100ml full-cream milk

Sauce:

25g unsalted butter
1 tbsp flour
150ml full-cream milk
1 tbsp fresh dill leaves, chopped
1 tbsp fresh chives
pinch of rock salt
finely ground black pepper

100g baby spinach leaves

- Place the haddock in an ovenproof dish and add the milk.

- Poach at the centre of a preheated oven at 180°C (gas mark 4) for about 20 minutes.

- At the same time, heat the butter in a medium saucepan and stir in the flour.

- Remove from the heat and gradually stir in the milk, stirring continuously.

- Stir in the dill and chives, season to taste and spoon the sauce over the smoked haddock fillets.

- At the same time, gently wilt the baby spinach leaves with 25g of butter in a medium saucepan.

- Serve the haddock over the baby spinach with sauce, and season to taste.

Carbohydrate content per serving: 2 grams

MEAT

Meat is healthy. Full stop. Organic meat provides all of the essential amino acids you need for health and many essential vitamins and minerals that are not present in foods of plant origin. That is not to say you need to eat meat: of course not, as all of those essential nutrients are also present in fish, shellfish and poultry (although red meat is by far the best source of iron). As previously described, 85 per cent of the cholesterol in your blood is made in your liver – not from meat in your diet – so consuming meat is not a significant factor in elevating blood cholesterol. The only reason to limit meat is because you should include fish, shellfish, poultry and veggies for a truly balanced – and delicious – diet.

Moroccan Lamb

SERVES 2

4 lamb steaks
1 tsp paprika
1 tsp ground cumin
½ tsp ground coriander
1 medium garlic clove, peeled and finely chopped
1 tbsp chopped fresh coriander leaves
2 tbsp extra-virgin olive oil
1 tsp mustard seeds, toasted

- Mix together the lamb steaks with the spices, garlic, coriander leaves and olive oil in a medium mixing bowl.

- Grill for about 4–5 minutes, turning once.

- Sprinkle with the toasted mustard seeds and serve.

Carbohydrate content per serving: 1 gram

Organic Beefburgers with Peppers and Mushrooms

SERVES 2

250g lean organic mince
2 shallots, peeled and diced
1 garlic clove, peeled and diced
1 tbsp extra-virgin olive oil
1 small red pepper, deseeded and sliced
100g button mushrooms, halved

- Mix together the mince, shallots, garlic and oil in a medium mixing bowl and season to taste. Form into 4 small burgers.

- Heat a little extra-virgin olive oil in a heavy-base grill pan and chargrill the pepper, mushrooms and burgers for about 5–6 minutes, turning the burgers once.

- Season to taste and serve.

Carbohydrate content per serving: 5 grams

Easy Sirloin Steak with Tomato Salsa

SERVES 2

3 large plum tomatoes
1 tbsp extra-virgin olive oil
2 medium sirloin steaks approximately 150g each
2 spring onions
1 tbsp balsamic vinegar
½ tbsp fresh oregano leaves, chopped
pinch of sea salt
freshly ground black pepper

- Place the tomatoes in a heat-proof bowl and cover with boiling water for 2 minutes.

- Drain and peel the tomatoes, remove the seeds and dice the flesh.

- Add 1 tbsp of extra-virgin olive oil to a medium frying pan and fry the steaks as required, approximately 2 minutes per side for rare, 3 minutes per side for medium, and 4 minutes per side for well done.

- Remove the steaks from the pan, cover and set aside.

- Add the tomato flesh, spring onion, balsamic vinegar, oregano and seasoning to the pan and heat through.

- Serve the steaks topped with tomato salsa.

Carbohydrate content per serving: 6 grams

Pan-fried Steak with Baked Halloumi

SERVES 2

1 tbsp extra-virgin olive oil
2 medium steaks, either rump or sirloin, approximately 150g each
2 beefsteak tomatoes, sliced
50g Halloumi cheese, sliced thinly
pinch of rock salt
freshly ground black pepper

- Heat the oil in a frying pan, add the steak and fry for about 5 minutes, turning once.

- At the same time, place the tomato slices in an ovenproof dish and top with the slices of Halloumi cheese.

- Bake the tomato and cheese in a preheated oven at 180°C (gas mark 4) for about 5 minutes.

- Serve the steak with the Halloumi and tomato and season to taste.

Carbohydrate content per serving: 3 grams

Marinated Pork Steaks

....

SERVES 2

3 tbsp extra-virgin olive oil
100ml dry red wine
1 tbsp red wine vinegar
1 garlic clove, peeled and chopped
2 shallots, peeled and diced
2 tbsp fresh rosemary, chopped
pinch of rock salt
freshly ground black pepper
2 medium pork steaks (about 150g each)
75g mangetout

- Mix together 1 tbsp of the olive oil, the red wine, wine vinegar, garlic, shallots and rosemary and season to taste.

- Pour the marinade over the pork steaks and place in the fridge for one hour.

- Add the remaining olive oil to a frying pan, add the pork steaks and fry for about 4 minutes per side, turning once.

- At the same time, lightly steam the mangetout for about 4–5 minutes.

Carbohydrate content per serving: 5 grams

Pork Steaks with Orange, Fennel and Rosemary

SERVES 2

2 medium pork steaks, approximately 150g each
½ tsp fennel seeds, crushed
2 tbsp freshly squeezed orange juice
1 garlic clove, peeled and chopped
1 tbsp rosemary, chopped
1 tbsp fresh oregano leaves, chopped (optional)

- Slice the pork steaks lengthways to create a pocket in each.
- Mix together the fennel seeds, orange juice, garlic, rosemary and oregano in a small mixing bowl.
- Spoon the mixture into the flap of each pork steak and bake in an ovenproof dish in the centre of a preheated oven at 180°C (gas mark 4) for about 30–35 minutes.
- Serve with Healthy Green Salad (see page 279).

Carbohydrate content per serving: 3 grams

Lamb Koftas

SERVES 2

300g lamb mince
2 shallots, peeled and finely chopped
1cm fresh ginger root, peeled and finely chopped
1 garlic clove, crushed
1 tsp ground turmeric
1 tsp ground cumin
1 tsp ground coriander
1 tbsp fresh mint leaves, finely chopped
1 egg, beaten
wooden skewers
100g natural yoghurt
1 tbsp fresh coriander leaves, finely chopped

- Add the lamb, shallots, ginger, garlic, spices, mint, and egg to a large mixing bowl, and combine thoroughly by hand.
- Soak the wooden skewers in cold water for 30 minutes before use.
- Mould the lamb koftas around the skewers and grill for about 6 minutes, turning frequently.
- Mix together the yoghurt and coriander leaves and chill.
- Serve the koftas with the chilled fresh yoghurt sauce.

Carbohydrate content per serving: 5 grams

Lean Lamb Chops with Herbs

SERVES 2

2 tbsp extra-virgin olive oil
1 shallot, peeled and diced
1 tbsp thyme leaves, chopped
1 tbsp oregano leaves, chopped
1 tbsp fresh flat-leaf parsley leaves, chopped
1 tbsp freshly squeezed lime juice
1 tbsp green peppercorns
2 large lamb chops

- Heat the extra-virgin olive oil in a medium frying pan, add the shallot and sauté for about 1 minute.
- Add the herbs and lime juice, then remove the mixture from the pan.
- Spoon the herb mixture on the chops and grill for about 15 minutes.
- Then grill for a further 15 minutes on the other side. Season to taste and serve with a mixed green salad (see page 281).

Carbohydrate content per serving: 2 grams

EGGS

As is the case with most 'natural' foods, eggs are high in nutrition and perfect for meals at any time of day. Scrambled eggs or omelettes are the ideal light meal, and can be combined with an almost limitless array of accompaniments, from spicy peppers and coriander in Mexican Scrambled Eggs, to Green Apple and Roquefort Omelette. Quick and easy to prepare with just a few tasty ingredients, satisfying and nutritious, eggs are the original 'fast' food.

Easy Omelette

SERVES 2

4 large free-range eggs
1 tbsp full-cream milk
pinch of sea salt
freshly ground black pepper
25g unsalted butter

- Beat the eggs in a medium mixing bowl, stirring in the milk and season to taste.

- Heat the butter in a medium omelette pan, add the mixture and cook on high for about 30 seconds, then reduce the heat.

- When the egg begins to set, fold the sides of the omelette to the centre and serve immediately.

Carbohydrate content per serving: 0–2 grams

Of course there are many potential fillings for omelette – you'll find lots of suggestions in the Mushroom Omelette recipe on page 274.

Mushroom Omelette

....

SERVES 2

omelette (see Easy Omelette, page 273)
25g butter
pinch of sea salt
freshly ground black pepper
50g button mushrooms, wiped and halved

- Prepare the Easy Omelette, as described.

- Heat the butter in a medium saucepan, add the mushrooms and sauté.

- As the omelette begins to set, spoon over the mushrooms, season to taste, fold over the omelette and serve.

> Carbohydrate content per serving: 5 grams

Mushrooms are just one delicious filling for omelettes – in fact the list is almost endless, such as:

- diced smoked salmon with chives
- asparagus and basil
- chopped fresh coriander
- Parma ham
- chives with plum tomato
- tomatoes with oregano

Green Apple and Roquefort Omelette

SERVES 2

2 tbsp butter
1 small apple, peeled, cored and sliced
4 large free-range eggs
2 tbsp Parmesan cheese, grated
50g Roquefort cheese, crumbled
pinch of sea salt
freshly ground black pepper

- Melt a tablespoon of butter in a medium omelette pan, add the apple slices and sauté for about 2 minutes.

- Remove the apple slices and melt the remaining tablespoon of butter in the pan.

- Add the eggs and, as the omelette begins to set, add the apple slices and the cheeses to the omelette and season to taste.

- Fold over the omelette and serve immediately.

Carbohydrate content per serving: 5 grams

Mexican Scrambled Eggs

SERVES 2

1 tbsp extra-virgin olive oil
2 shallots, peeled and finely chopped
2 garlic cloves, peeled and finely chopped
1 tsp ground cumin
2 medium plum tomatoes, finely chopped
1 small red pepper, deseeded and finely chopped
1 medium green pepper, deseeded and finely chopped

For the eggs:
1 tbsp butter
4 large free-range eggs, beaten
1 tbsp coriander leaves, chopped
2 tbsp freshly grated Parmesan cheese

- Heat the olive oil in a medium frying pan, add the shallots and garlic and sauté for 2–3 minutes

- Stir in the cumin, tomatoes and peppers and cook for about 3–4 minutes. Season to taste and set aside.

- At the same time, heat the butter in a small saucepan.

- Stir in the eggs and stir gently until they begin to set.

- Stir the eggs into the tomato mixture, add the coriander and heat through.

- Serve immediately, topped with Parmesan cheese.

Carbohydrate content per serving: 14 grams

SALADS

Salads have travelled a long way since the days of a few wilted lettuce leaves with soggy tomatoes. A salad can easily make a satisfying and healthy main meal in itself, such as Spicy Venison with Coriander Salad, or an accompaniment to a light lunch or dinner, such as the ubiquitous Healthy Green Salad. And, to enjoy salads to the maximum, make your own dressing; nothing could be simpler if you adhere to the simple formula of 1 tbsp wine vinegar to 5 tbsp extra-virgin olive oil (plus seasoning) – and the potential variations are immense. Always add vinaigrette or mayonnaise to a salad as the healthy fats in the dressing slow the digestion of the salad ingredients, releasing the energy from the meal slowly. We have also included a recipe for Provençal Sauce – cooled, it provides the perfect dressing for chicken and salads.

Lebanese Cucumber Salad

SERVES 2

2 Lebanese cucumbers, sliced thinly
50ml crème fraîche
1 tbsp white wine vinegar
1 tbsp chopped fresh dill
1 tbsp chopped fresh chives
pinch of sea salt
freshly ground black pepper

- Mix the ingredients together in a large mixing bowl and serve chilled.

Carbohydrate content per serving: 4 grams

Spicy Venison with Coriander Salad

SERVES 2

2 venison medallion steaks, approximately 150g each
2 medium plum tomatoes, sliced
100g wild rocket leaves
1 Lebanese cucumber, thinly sliced

Dressing:

1 tbsp lime juice
1 tbsp fish sauce
1 garlic clove, peeled and chopped
1 small green chilli, deseeded and finely chopped
1 tbsp fresh coriander leaves, chopped

- Place the venison steaks on a baking tray and cook in a preheated oven at 180°C (gas mark 4) for about 25 minutes.

- Remove from the oven and set aside to cool.

- Slice the venison steaks thinly.

- Combine the tomatoes, rocket and cucumber in a large bowl and add the venison.

- Whisk the ingredients of the dressing in a small bowl.

- Drizzle the dressing over the salad and serve.

Carbohydrate content per serving: 8 grams

Healthy Green Salad

SERVES 2

100g French beans, trimmed
100g snow peas, trimmed
100g sugar snap peas, trimmed
2 tbsp fresh basil leaves
2 tbsp fresh flat-leaf parsley leaves
100g wild rocket
sprigs of parsley, to garnish

Dressing:

1 tbsp Dijon mustard
1 tbsp lime juice
1 tbsp extra-virgin olive oil

- Steam the French beans, snow peas and sugar snap peas for about 10 minutes, rinse under cold water and drain.
- Add the beans and peas to a large mixing bowl with the basil, parsley leaves and rocket.
- Whisk the ingredients of the dressing in a small bowl.
- Drizzle over the dressing and toss the salad.

Carbohydrate content per serving: 8 grams

Grilled Asparagus with Italian-style Sauce

SERVES 2

6 cherry tomatoes, halved
1 garlic clove, peeled and finely chopped
6 tbsp lime juice
2 tbsp basil leaves
25g butter
2 tbsp oregano leaves
300g asparagus, trimmed
100g baby spinach leaves
10 black olives

- Cook the tomato, garlic and lime juice over a high heat for 1–2 minutes.

- Reduce the heat and simmer for about 3–4 minutes.

- Stir in the herbs, simmer gently for about another minute, then set aside to cool.

- Melt the butter in a small saucepan, brush the asparagus with the melted butter and grill under a hot grill, no closer than 15cm from the grill, for 8–10 minutes, turning once.

- Arrange the spinach leaves on the serving plates, top with asparagus and olives, and drizzle over the Italian-style sauce.

Carbohydrate content per serving: 8 grams

Mixed Green Salad with Thyme and Mustard Dressing

SERVES 2

100g wild rocket leaves
100g watercress
50g mangetout, topped and tailed and sliced on the diagonal
1 Lebanese cucumber, sliced lengthwise
1 tbsp lemon juice
1 tbsp fish sauce
1 tsp brown sugar
Thyme and Mustard Dressing (see page 300)

- Toss the ingredients of the salad in a large mixing bowl.
- Drizzle over the dressing and serve.

Carbohydrate content per serving: 3 grams

Kiwi Fruit and Lime Salad

SERVES 2

3 kiwi fruit, peeled and sliced
10 green grapes
1 tbsp fresh mint leaves
2 tbsp freshly squeezed lime juice

- Mix together the ingredients and serve immediately.

Carbohydrate content per serving: 12 grams

Feta Salad

SERVES 2

100g feta cheese, cubed
8 vine-ripened cherry tomatoes, halved
1 Lebanese cucumber, sliced vertically
10 black olives
1 tbsp lime juice
1 tbsp extra-virgin olive oil
pinch of sea salt
freshly ground black pepper
1 tbsp freshly grated Parmesan cheese

- Toss the salad ingredients together in a salad mixing bowl and season to taste.
- Sprinkle with freshly grated Parmesan cheese and serve.

Carbohydrate content per serving: 4 grams

Provençal Sauce

SERVES 2

1 tbsp extra-virgin olive oil
2 shallots, peeled and diced
2 garlic cloves, crushed
400g can plum tomatoes
1 tsp tarragon leaves
1 tsp fresh flat-leaf parsley leaves
pinch of rock salt
freshly ground black pepper

- Heat the olive oil in a medium frying pan and sauté the shallots and garlic for about 2–3 minutes.

- Drain the tomatoes and set aside the juice.
- Stir in the tomatoes, tarragon and parsley, and season to taste.
- Stir in the juice from the tomatoes and simmer for about 30 minutes.
- Set aside to cool before serving.

Carbohydrate content per serving: 7 grams

Walnut, Herb and Vegetable Medley

SERVES 2

3 tbsp extra-virgin olive oil
1 courgette, sliced julienne
1 carrot, peeled and sliced julienne
1 small leek, sliced into thin strips
50g walnuts
1 shallot, peeled and diced
1 tbsp coriander leaves, chopped
1 tbsp flat-leaf parsley, chopped
pinch of sea salt
freshly ground black pepper

- Heat the extra-virgin olive oil in a medium frying pan
- Stir-fry the courgette, carrot, leek, walnuts, shallot and herbs for about 3–4 minutes
- Season to taste and serve immediately

Carbohydrate content per serving: 7 grams

VEGGIES

Oven-baked Ricotta with Vine-ripened Cherry Tomatoes

SERVES 2

2 tbsp extra-virgin olive oil
1 tbsp pine nuts
1 garlic clove, peeled and chopped
100g watercress
150g ricotta cheese
1 egg, beaten
1 tbsp basil leaves, chopped
200g vine cherry tomatoes
1 tbsp balsamic vinegar
freshly ground black pepper

- Heat 1 tbsp olive oil in a medium frying pan, add the pine nuts and garlic and sauté for about 2 minutes.

- Add the watercress and cook for about 20 seconds. Allow to cool.

- Add the cheese, egg and basil, mix and pour into a pre-prepared baking dish.

- Roast for 15 minutes in a preheated oven at 200°C (gas mark 6).

- At the same time, add the tomatoes, vinegar and remaining oil to a small baking dish and roast uncovered for about 15 minutes.

- Serve the roast ricotta with the tomatoes and season to taste.

Carbohydrate content per serving: 4 grams

Cheese and Spinach Bake

SERVES 2

300g fresh baby spinach leaves, washed and stems removed
150g ricotta cheese
75g feta cheese, crumbled
2 egg whites
1 tbsp fresh basil leaves, chopped
1 tbsp freshly squeezed lemon juice
pinch of sea salt
freshly ground black pepper

- Mix together the spinach, ricotta cheese, feta cheese, egg whites, basil and lemon juice in a medium mixing bowl.
- Add the mixture to an ovenproof dish and cook in the centre of a preheated oven at 180°C (gas mark 4) for about 1 hour.
- Season to taste and serve.

Carbohydrate content per serving: 6 grams

Oven-baked Aubergine

....

SERVES 2

1 large aubergine
1 tsp sea salt
2 eggs, beaten
1 tbsp butter
freshly ground black pepper
1 small shallot, peeled and diced
1 tbsp fresh oregano leaves
2 large plum tomatoes, sliced thinly
50g Emmental cheese, grated
25g Parmesan cheese, grated
pinch of paprika

- Peel and slice the aubergine. Place the slices in a medium sauce-pan with some salt and cover with boiling water.

- Leave in the boiling water for about 10 minutes and drain.

- Mash the aubergine and stir in the eggs, butter, pepper, shallots and oregano.

- Line a baking dish with greaseproof paper and cover the bottom with the tomato slices.

- Top with the aubergine mixture and sprinkle over the grated Emmental and Parmesan cheese.

- Add a pinch of paprika and bake in a preheated oven at 180°C (gas mark 4) for about 40 minutes.

Carbohydrate content per serving: 10 grams

Goats' Cheese with Chervil and Parsley

SERVES 2

200g fresh goats' cheese
1 tbsp fresh parsley leaves, chopped
1 tbsp fresh chervil (or chives)
1 small shallot, peeled and diced
4 capers (optional)
4 black peppercorns
pinch of rock salt
½ tsp white wine vinegar
1 tsp lemon juice
½ tsp extra-virgin olive oil

- Mix the cheese with the chopped fresh herbs, shallot, capers and peppercorns and season to taste.
- Stir in the vinegar, lemon juice and olive oil.
- Spoon the cheese mixture into two small ramekins and place in the fridge for about 1–2 hours.
- Serve with Healthy Green Salad (see page 279).

Carbohydrate content per serving: 2 grams

Skewered Halloumi and Pepper Kebabs

SERVES 2

3 courgettes, chopped on the diagonal
1 medium red pepper, deseeded and quartered
1 medium yellow pepper, deseeded and quartered
100g Halloumi cheese, cubed
50g unsalted butter
2 tbsp dry white wine
1 tbsp fresh basil leaves, chopped
1 tbsp fresh chives, snipped

- Alternate the courgette, pepper and Halloumi pieces on skewers.
- Melt the butter, add the wine and herbs and gently sauté for about 1 minute. Brush the kebabs with the herb-and-butter mixture and grill for about 8 minutes, turning once. Season to taste and serve immediately.

Carbohydrate content per serving: 6 grams

Steamed Veggies with Fresh Ginger Dressing

SERVES 2

1 small cauliflower, florets only
100g mangetout, trimmed
2 tbsp extra-virgin olive oil
1 tbsp freshly squeezed lime juice
pinch of sea salt
freshly ground black pepper
3cm root ginger, peeled and grated
1 tbsp fresh basil leaves, chopped

- Boil the cauliflower florets in salted water for about 2 minutes.

- Stir in the mangetout and cook for a further 2 minutes, then drain and rinse with cold water.

- In a small bowl, mix together the extra-virgin olive oil, lime juice, salt and pepper and ginger. Stir in the basil, then toss the dressing with the vegetables.

- Serve immediately.

Carbohydrate content per serving: 4 grams

Roasted Veggie Fusion

SERVES 2

1 large courgette, sliced on the diagonal
1 yellow pepper, deseeded and sliced thinly
1 fennel bulb, sliced finely
3 cherry tomatoes, halved
1 tbsp extra-virgin olive oil
2 tbsp lime juice
1 tbsp oregano leaves, chopped

- Place the vegetables on a baking tray, and drizzle over the olive oil.

- Cook in a preheated oven at 180°C (gas mark 4) for about 20–25 minutes.

- Drizzle over the lime juice and garnish with oregano leaves.

Carbohydrate content per serving: 9 grams

Garlic Mushrooms

SERVES 2

1 tbsp extra-virgin olive oil
100g shiitake mushrooms
100g chestnut mushrooms
100g brown mushrooms
3 garlic cloves, peeled and finely chopped
3 egg yolks, beaten
freshly ground black pepper
1 tbsp fresh oregano leaves

- Heat the extra-virgin olive oil in a large frying pan, stir in the mushrooms and garlic and sauté for about 4–5 minutes.

- Stir in the egg yolks and cook until set (about 2 minutes).

- Season to taste and add the fresh oregano leaves.

- Serve immediately.

Carbohydrate content per serving: 1 gram

Artichoke Hearts with Vegetables

....

SERVES 2

1 tbsp extra-virgin olive oil
1 shallot, peeled and sliced
1 carrot, peeled and sliced
1 celery stick, trimmed and sliced on the diagonal into 2-cm lengths
1 garlic clove, peeled and sliced
100ml vegetable stock
50ml dry white wine
100g fresh peas
200g jar artichoke hearts, drained
1 tbsp fresh basil leaves, chopped
freshly ground black pepper

- Heat the extra-virgin olive oil in a medium saucepan, add the shallot, carrot and celery and braise for 2–3 minutes.

- Stir in the garlic and cook for a further 2 minutes.

- Add the vegetable stock and wine and simmer for 10–15 minutes.

- Stir in the peas and artichoke hearts and heat through for a further 3–4 minutes.

- Add the basil, season to taste and serve immediately.

Carbohydrate content per serving: 5 grams

Mushroom Stroganoff

SERVES 2

50g unsalted butter
2 shallots, peeled and sliced
100g chestnut mushrooms, wiped and sliced
100g shiitake mushrooms, wiped and sliced
100g brown mushrooms, wiped and sliced
5g dried porcini mushrooms, soaked
150ml dry white wine
100ml sour cream
freshly ground black pepper

- Melt the butter in a large frying pan, add the shallots and sauté for 5–7 minutes.

- Remove the shallots from the frying pan and set aside to cool.

- Add the mushrooms to the pan and sauté for 2–3 minutes.

- Return the shallots to the pan, add the wine and season to taste.

- Simmer for about 10 minutes.

- Stir in the sour cream and serve with a green salad.

Carbohydrate content per serving: 7 grams

Roasted Red Sweet Peppers with Capers and Oregano

....

SERVES 2

4 red sweet peppers, halved lengthways and deseeded
1 tbsp extra-virgin olive oil
2 garlic cloves, peeled and chopped
1 tbsp capers, drained and rinsed
1 tbsp fresh oregano leaves, chopped
pinch of sea salt
freshly ground black pepper

- Place the peppers on a medium baking dish, with the open side uppermost, drizzle over the oil and sprinkle with garlic.
- Bake the peppers in a preheated oven at 200°C (gas mark 6) for 15–20 minutes.
- Add the capers and oregano to the peppers and return to the oven for 2–3 minutes.
- Season to taste and serve.

Carbohydrate content per serving: 7 grams

Pea purée

SERVES 2

200g fresh peas (or frozen if necessary)
½ tsp cumin seeds
½ tsp coriander seeds
1 tbsp extra-virgin olive oil
1 tbsp freshly squeezed lemon juice
1 tbsp fresh basil leaves, chopped
1 green chilli, deseeded and finely chopped
pinch of rock salt
freshly ground black pepper

- Add the peas to medium saucepan with boiling water and simmer for 4–5 minutes.

- Rinse in a colander under cold water and set aside.

- Crush the cumin and coriander seeds with a pestle and mortar and then place the peas, crushed coriander and cumin seeds, olive oil, lemon juice, basil leaves and green chilli in a blender and blend for 2 minutes.

- Season to taste and set aside in the fridge to cool.

Carbohydrate content per serving: 5 grams

Kale with Pine Nuts and Sunflower Seeds

SERVES 2

1 tbsp extra-virgin olive oil
2 shallots, peeled and chopped
1 garlic clove, peeled and chopped
2cm root ginger, peeled and finely chopped
200g kale leaves, trimmed and chopped
100ml vegetable stock
25g toasted pine nuts
25g sunflower seeds
freshly ground black pepper

- Heat the extra-virgin olive oil in a large frying pan, add the shallots and sauté for 2–3 minutes.

- Add the garlic, ginger and kale and sauté for 3–4 minutes.

- Add the stock and simmer for 8–9 minutes.

- Remove from the heat, stir in the pine nuts and sunflower seeds, season and serve.

Carbohydrate content per serving: 3 grams

Roasted Pepper, Aubergine and Halloumi

SERVES 2

1 small red pepper
1 small yellow pepper
1 medium aubergine, sliced thinly
100g Halloumi, cut into 2–3-cm slices
2 tsp lemon zest
1 tbsp extra-virgin olive oil
1 tbsp flat-leaf parsley, chopped
1 tbsp mint leaves, chopped
3 tbsp freshly squeezed lemon juice
freshly ground black pepper

- Place the peppers under a hot grill and cook for 10–15 minutes, then set aside to cool.

- When the peppers have cooled, remove the skin, and slice the peppers thickly.

- If you have time, you can salt the aubergine before cooking to remove any bitterness: place the aubergine slices in a colander and sprinkle with salt, leave for 30 minutes and then rinse in fresh water.

- Dry the aubergine with kitchen roll.

- Place the aubergine slices on a baking tray, brush with olive oil and cook under a hot grill for 3–4 minutes, turning once, then set aside.

- Place the Halloumi under the hot grill and cook for 2–3 minutes per side turning once.

- Mix together lemon zest and 1 tbsp extra-virgin olive oil in a small bowl.

- In a medium mixing bowl, add the peppers to the aubergine,

Halloumi, flat-leaf parsley and mint, add the lemon juice and lemon zest.

- Season to taste and serve.

Carbohydrate content per serving: 9 grams

Roast Mixed-pepper Salad

SERVES 2

1 medium red pepper
1 medium orange pepper
1 medium green pepper
2 tsp balsamic vinegar
1 tbsp extra-virgin olive oil
1 tbsp honey
1 tsp capers, rinsed
1 tbsp pine nuts
1 tbsp flat-leaf parsley

- Preheat the grill to high, place the peppers on the grill tray (no closer than 8–10 cm from the element) and grill for about 15 minutes, turning once.

- Set aside to cool.

- In a small bowl, mix together the balsamic vinegar, extra-virgin olive oil, honey and capers.

- When the peppers have cooled, remove the skins and slice the peppers into thick slices.

- Place the peppers in a large bowl and toss with dressing.

- Add the pine nuts and parsley, season to taste and serve.

Carbohydrate content per serving: 7 grams

DIPS AND DRESSINGS

Dips and dressings are usually of the ready-prepared variety and have the unfortunate reputation of being time-consuming and difficult to make. Nothing could be further from the truth. As you will see, dips and dressings are quick and simple to prepare – and are much more tasty and nutritious than their ready-prepared counterparts. Here are a few delicious starters – but the list of potential combinations is almost endless.

Smoked-salmon Dip

SERVES 2

100g smoked salmon, diced
100g cream cheese
1 tsp freshly squeezed lemon juice
1 spring onion, diced
1 tbsp fresh flat-leaf parsley
1 small garlic clove, peeled and diced
pinch of rock salt
freshly ground black pepper

• Add the ingredients to a blender and blend until smooth, then set aside to chill.

Carbohydrate content per serving: 3 grams

Spicy Chickpea and Red Pepper Dip

SERVES 2

175g can chickpeas, drained
300g jar sweet red peppers, drained

1 tbsp extra-virgin olive oil
1 shallot, peeled and diced
1 green chilli, deseeded and diced
1 garlic clove, peeled and diced
1 tsp freshly squeezed lime juice
pinch of sea salt
freshly ground black pepper

- Blend the chickpeas, peppers, extra-virgin olive oil, shallot, chilli, garlic and lime juice.

- Season to taste and chill before serving.

Carbohydrate content per serving: 16 grams

Hot Crab Dip with Crudités

SERVES 2

200g fresh white crab meat
50ml crème fraîche
100g cream cheese
1 tbsp freshly squeezed lime juice
1 small shallot, peeled and diced
5–6 drops Tabasco sauce
pinch of sea salt
1 tbsp chopped fresh dill

- Mix the ingredients together in a medium bowl and set aside to chill.

- Serve with crudités.

Carbohydrate content per serving: 3 grams

Herb Dressing

SERVES 2

2 tbsp spearmint leaves
2 tbsp coriander leaves
2 thin slices of ginger root, sliced finely
2 tbsp lime juice
1 tbsp extra-virgin olive oil

• Whisk together the ingredients of the dressing in a small bowl.

Carbohydrate content per serving: 2 grams

Thyme and Mustard Dressing

SERVES 2

1 tbsp lime juice
1 tbsp white wine vinegar
1 tbsp American mustard
1 tbsp water
2 tbsp fresh lemon thyme leaves, chopped
2 tbsp extra-virgin olive oil

• Whisk together the ingredients in a small bowl.

Carbohydrate content per serving: 2 grams

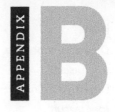

Snacks to Avoid

Snacking on biscuits, cakes and pastries during the working day can be extremely detrimental to your health, by increasing the blood-sugar concentration and increasing your risk of diabetes, high blood pressure and heart disease. Obviously, all brands vary in shape and size, so that the table can be only be an approximation, but this places the subject in perspective. Selecting crisps, biscuits or pastries from the office tea trolley, stopping off at the local shop while travelling to work, or the kiosk at the railway station or the local garage – all are potential sources of problems.

Biscuits, cakes and pastries

Item	Carbs (grams) per 100g (and per unit as applicable)	Calories
Chocolate-chip	70	500
(per biscuit)	7	50
Chocolate-coated	70	520
(per biscuit)	16	130

→

Item	Carbs (grams) per 100g (and per unit as applicable)	Calories
Digestive chocolate	70	500
(per biscuit)	10	75
Digestive plain	65	450
(per biscuit)	10	70
Flapjack	57	475
(per biscuit)	13	110
Ginger	80	450
(per biscuit)	8	45
Jaffa Cake	70	370
(per biscuit)	10	20
Kit Kat	60	506
(per biscuit)	12	106
Shortbread	65	500
(per biscuit)	10	80

Crackers and crispbreads

Cream cracker	65	450
(per biscuit)	5	30
Oatcakes	65	450
(per biscuit)	6	45
Wholemeal cracker	75	420
(per biscuit)	5	30

Cakes

Banana	70	420
(per slice 50g)	35	210
Carrot	45	400
(per slice 50g)	23	200
Carrot & orange	55	440
(per slice 50g)	15	122
Cheesecake	33	310
(per slice 50g)	15	155
Cherry	60	400
(per slice 50g)	30	200

Item	Carbs (grams) per 100g (and per unit as applicable)	Calories
Chocolate	60	400
(per slice 50g)	30	200
Chocolate éclair	35	380
(per slice 50g)	25	270
Doughnut	50	340
Fruitcake	50	320
(per slice 50g)	25	160
Gateau	45	350
(per slice 50g)	23	175
Ice fruit bun	45	300
(per slice 50g)	33	225
Madeira	60	400
(per slice 50g)	30	200
Mud cake	60	420
(per slice 50g)	30	210
Sponge cake	60	350
(per slice 50g)	30	175

Pastries

Croissant	40	350
(per croissant)	25	210

Danish

Apple Danish	45	300
Blueberry Danish	40	300
Chocolate Danish	25	300

Bread

Item	Carbs (grams) per 100g	Calories
Bagel	30	140
Baguette	23	130
Focaccia	30	140
Hamburger roll	40	215

→

Item	Carbs (grams) per 100g	Calories
Naan	50	340
Pita	20–50	50–230
Tortilla	15–25	70–150

Cereals

Item	Carbs (grams) per 100g	Calories
Bran flakes	70	320
Cornflakes	85	360
Fibre-and-fruit flakes	75	350
Cheerios	70	372
Porridge oats	73	400

Dips, popcorn and crisps

Item	Carbs (grams) per 100g (and per unit as applicable)	Calories
Salsa dip	9	40
Garlic-and-herb dip	7	370
Popcorn	70	470
Potato crisps:		
ready-salted	48	544
(per packet)	12	156
salt & vinegar	45	550
(per packet)	11	140
tomato	45	550
(per packet)	12	140

Chocolate

Item	Carbs (grams) per 100g	Calories
Caramel whip	52	435
Flake	56	530
Mars bar	70	450
Milk	60	520
Maltesers	61	480
Milky Way	72	450

Sweets

Item	Carbs (grams) per 100g (and per unit as applicable)	Calories
Chewing gum:		
sugar-free	less than 1	40
(per piece)	less than 1	4
normal	30	100
(per piece)	3	10

Drinks

Item	Carbs (grams) per 100g	Calories
Beer	30	320
Coffee, black	1	1
Coffee, cappuccino	10	134
Coffee, white	3	25
Fruit juice	8	25
Lemonade	18	74
Orange	8	33
Milk shakes:		
chocolate	20	120
strawberry	20	120
Port	6	25
Sherry	6	60
Rosé wine	3	75
White wine	6	99
Red wine	3	90

Index